Assisted Living Through Research, Policy, and Practice

Helena Temkin-Greener · Sheryl Zimmerman
Editors

Assisted Living Through Research, Policy, and Practice

What's in the Name?

Springer

Editors
Helena Temkin-Greener
School of Medicine and Dentistry
Department of Public Health Sciences
University of Rochester
Rochester, NY, USA

Sheryl Zimmerman
Center for Excellence in Assisted Living
(CEAL@UNC), School of Social Work,
and the Cecil G. Sheps Center for Health
Services Research
University of North Carolina
Chapel Hill, NC, USA

ISBN 978-3-032-32087-2 ISBN 978-3-032-32088-9 (eBook)
https://doi.org/10.1007/978-3-032-32088-9

This Springer imprint is published by the registered company Springer Nature Switzerland AG
The registered company address is: Gewerbestrasse 11, 6330 Cham, Switzerland

Preface

The promise of assisted living has long captured the imagination of providers, policymakers, families, and older adults themselves. Marketed as a middle path between independent living and nursing home care, the assisted living philosophy is to deliver personalized "assistance" while preserving the dignity, autonomy, and quality of "living" that define a meaningful later life. As the US population ages and the demand for such settings continues to grow, questions persist: To what extent do these communities truly fulfill that dual promise? Do they provide services and supports that empower residents to live with purpose and maximum independence, or do workforce, regulatory, and operational realities sometimes limit the very quality of life they aim to protect?

This edited volume brings together leading scholars, practitioners, consumers, and other experts to examine assisted living through a multifaceted lens. Each chapter explores a distinct dimension—ranging from regulatory frameworks and workforce availability to residents' daily experiences, mental health, dementia care, end-of-life considerations, and quality—offering evidence-based insights drawn from research as well as the perspectives of providers and consumers. Collectively, the contributions interrogate the central research question that drives the book: **To what extent does today's assisted living deliver on its foundational promise to provide meaningful assistance while enabling authentic living?**

The idea for this collection emerged from ongoing conversations in the fields of gerontology, long-term care policy, and health services research, as the rapid expansion of assisted living outpaced comprehensive, integrated analysis. While individual studies have illuminated specific aspects of the field, there has been little synthesis of the broad range of research under a unifying question. This book aims to fill that gap, providing a resource for researchers, policymakers, administrators, clinicians, and advocates seeking to understand both the achievements and the shortcomings of assisted living as it exists today—and, hopefully, to inform improvements for tomorrow.

We are deeply grateful to the chapter authors for their thoughtful contributions, rigorous scholarship, and commitment to advancing this important dialogue. Their diverse expertise—from regulatory analysis to resident-centered qualitative research—has immeasurably enriched the volume and the field of assisted living itself. Special thanks are extended to the Springer Nature editorial team for their guidance and support throughout the process.

It is our hope that this book will stimulate reflection, spark debate, and ultimately contribute to the evolution of assisted living into a model that more fully honors the promise of assistance with genuine living.

Rochester, NY, USA
Chapel Hill, NC, USA
March 2026

Helena Temkin-Greener
Sheryl Zimmerman

Contents

Editors and Contributors

About the Editors

Helena Temkin-Greener is Professor Emeritus in the Department of Public Health Sciences at the University of Rochester, School of Medicine and Dentistry, in New York, USA. She is also the founder and the director of the Program of All-Inclusive Care for the Elderly (PACE) National Data Center (PDAC). Her research is focused in the following areas: quality of care—developing outcome measures and assessing quality of care in community-based, hospital and long-term care settings; organizational performance—developing and validating measures of care process, teamwork, and patient safety; aging and long-term care—assessing the impact of individual and organizational risk factors on quality of care for vulnerable elderly, including disparities; palliative and end-of-life care—design, implementation and evaluation of interventions to improve care; mental illness—understanding access to and quality of care for patients with mental health disorders and with dementia. Her work has been funded by the National Institutes of Health, the Agency for Healthcare Research and Quality, PCORI, and other federal and private funders. She is the co-editor of this book and a co-author of Chapters 1 and 3.

Sheryl Zimmerman is a University Distinguished Professor in the School of Social Work, the Executive Director of the Center for Excellence in Assisted Living at the University of North Carolina (CEAL@UNC), and Co-Director of the Program on Aging, Chronic Illness, and Long-term Care in the Cecil G. Sheps Center for Health Services Research at the University of North Carolina at Chapel Hill, USA. She is internationally recognized as a leader in research related to care and outcomes for older adults receiving long-term care, including persons living with dementia. In 1996 Zimmerman founded the Collaborative Studies of Long-Term Care, the largest ongoing national research consortium of thousands of long-term care settings across the country that have participated in almost 100 projects with continuous funding from the National Institutes of Health, the Agency for Healthcare Research and Quality, and foundations. She has written five books and more than 450 peer-reviewed publications. She is the co-editor of this book and a co-author of Chapters 1, 5, and 10.

Contributors

Ijebusonma Agundu is a Behavioral Health Counselor at Boston Children's Hospital in Massachusetts, USA, and a public health specialist focused on equitable care. She leads opioid prevention efforts designing evidence-based interventions that integrate behavioral health, chronic disease, and health education. She uses electronic medical records to improve care coordination and applies mixed-methods research to strengthen prevention strategies. She is the co-author of Chapter 6.

Rita Altman is Principal Owner of Rita Altman Memory Care Consulting LLC, located in Mechanicsburg, Pennsylvania, USA. She has more than 40 years of nursing experience which includes nursing education, intergenerational programming, management in childcare, adult day care, and executive-level leadership in assisted living and memory care. She is the co-author of Chapter 10.

David Balter is pursuing a Master's degree in Social Work at the University of North Carolina at Chapel Hill, USA. He is a contributing author to Chapter 5.

Emmanuelle Belanger is an Associate Professor of Health Services, Policy & Practice at the Center for Gerontology and Healthcare Research within Brown University's School of Public Health in Rhode Island, USA. Trained in both social and health sciences, she earned her Ph.D. from McGill University in the Departments of Psychiatry and Family Medicine. Dr. Belanger has led a research program using mixed-methods approaches, focused on assessing and managing patient-reported symptoms in older adults, improving the quality of end-of-life care across diverse settings, and examining decision-making processes around palliative care. She is the author of Chapter 8.

Thomas Caprio is Professor and an academic geriatrician and serves as hospice/palliative care physician at the University of Rochester Medical Center in New York, USA. He is the Chief Medical Officer for UR Medicine Home Care and is the Hospice Medical Director. Dr. Caprio is a national leader in geriatrics and gerontology education, as well as a leader in research focusing on home health care, assisted living, nursing homes, and end-of-life care. He is the director of the Finger Lakes Geriatric Education Center (FLGEC) at the University of Rochester where he oversees the development and implementation of regional, state, and national education and training programs to support the health care workforce and family caregivers. He has received numerous awards recognizing his accomplishments and advocacy efforts, as well as federal, state, and foundation grant funding to support his work. He has published over 100 articles, book chapters, and white papers. He is the co-author of Chapter 7.

Wenhan Guo is Assistant Professor in the Department of Social and Public Health at Ohio University in Athens, Ohio, USA. His research focuses on aging, long-term care, post-acute care, hospice, and health disparities, with a particular interest in improving outcomes for vulnerable populations. He uses large-scale administrative and survey data to examine care delivery, workforce policy, and regulatory environments in long-term care settings. His work aims to inform evidence-based policy and improve equity and quality for vulnerable populations across healthcare systems. He is the co-author of Chapter 3.

Sarah Howd is Assistant Professor of Medicine and Geriatrics at the University of Rochester in New York, USA. She is a geriatrician and serves as the Associate Medical Director of the Senior Living Practice of the University of Rochester Medicine Geriatrics Group. She cares for patients at several area independent and assisted living communities. She is a certified medical director and serves as medical director of seven assisted living communities. Dr. Howd was a Tideswell Emerging Leader in Aging Scholar in 2022 through the University of California at San Francisco (UCSF) and the American Geriatric Society. She recently served as the Chair of AMDA's national subcommittee for Assisted Living. She is the co-author of Chapter 7.

Cassandra L. Hua is Assistant Professor in the Department of Public Health, Zuckerberg College of Health Sciences, University of Massachusetts, Lowell, Massachusetts, USA. She is a health services researcher working to help inform policies and practices that improve the quality of long-term care services and supports for older adults. In addition to a broad background in gerontology, she has expertise in conducting analyses using secondary data, survey data, and large administrative datasets such as Medicare claims. Her research focuses on regulatory and organizational characteristics related to the quality of care provided to assisted living residents, especially those with dementia. She is the co-author of Chapter 6.

Candace L. Kemp is a Professor of Gerontology at Georgia State University, USA, and has an appointment in the Department of Sociology. Dr. Kemp's research examines long-term care arrangements, partnerships, networks, and experiences, including ethics; dementia care; meaningful engagement; and end-of-life experiences from the perspectives of older adults and their myriad of paid and unpaid care partners. Much of her research is funded by the National Institute on Aging (NIA) at the National Institutes of Health (NIH) and seeks to improve quality of life for older adults and those who support them. She is the author of Chapter 9.

Walter Moczygemba is the Manager of the national Center for Excellence in Assisted Living at the University of North Carolina at Chapel Hill (CEAL@UNC), USA. He has more than a decade of experience in dementia and long-term care, including providing direct care as a Program Director at a nonprofit adult day center, clinical experience as a social work intern at a Veterans Health Administration Geriatric Research Education and Clinical Center, and as an ongoing consultant with the Alzheimer's Association. His work at CEAL@UNC focuses on advancing well-being for those who live and work in assisted living through research, practice, and policy. He is the co-author of Chapter 10.

Elizabeth Morton is a graduate student pursuing her MD degree at the University of North Carolina School of Medicine, Chapel Hill, USA. She is a contributing author to Chapter 5.

Lindsay B. Schwartz is the Founder and Principal at Workforce & Quality Innovations (WQI), LLC, a consulting, research, and advisory firm which she started in 2022. She is a nationally recognized expert on quality in assisted living, measure development, and workforce issues in long-term care. Prior to starting WQI, Dr. Schwartz was an Associate Vice President of Workforce and Quality Improvement for the American Health Care Association/National Center for Assisted Living (AHCA/NCAL). During her tenure at AHCA/NCAL, she developed and implemented quality-improvement initiatives, developed quality measures, and oversaw workforce initiatives for the association. Dr. Schwartz was part of the development team for the CoreQ, a set of customer-satisfaction measures for long-term care settings. She led the process for National Quality Forum (NQF) endorsement for the assisted living CoreQ measures, the first AL-specific measures to be endorsed by NQF. She was lead on COVID-19 workforce issues including Occupational Safety and Health Administration (OSHA) compliance. She is the author of Chapter 4.

Philip D. Sloane is Professor of Family Medicine and Geriatrics at the University of North Carolina at Chapel Hill, USA, where he co-directs the Program on Aging, Chronic Illness, and Long-Term Care of the Cecil G. Sheps Center for Health Services Research. His clinical work has included community practice, nursing home medical directorship, rural emergency department work, and staffing a Program of All-Inclusive Care for the Elderly. As a researcher, his work has included over 50 funded studies, most of which have focused on understanding and improving health services and care for older persons, particularly those with Alzheimer's disease and related disorders. He is particularly noted for his work around the management of behavioral expressions in persons with Alzheimer's disease, for which he received the prestigious Pioneer Award from the US Alzheimer's Association. He is the co-author of Chapter 5.

Jennifer Svoboda is an assisted living Operator for Sapphire Health Services based out of Portland, Oregon, USA. She has been working in long-term care since 1994 starting as a social worker and consultant. She moved into the assisted living side of the profession in 2008 first as an Executive Director, then to leadership roles at the regional level. She sits on several American Health Care Association (AHCA) and National Center for Assisted Living (NCAL) committees, is an At-Large Member of the NCAL board, and is the Board Chair of the Nevada Health Care Association. She is the co-author of Chapter 10.

Jinjiao Wang is Professor and Assistant Dean for Research at the University of Texas Health Science Center, School of Nursing, in San Antonio, Texas, USA. Dr. Wang is a nurse scientist, educator, and innovator dedicated to transforming home- and community-based care for older adults. Her interdisciplinary research bridges clinical relevance with systems innovation, advancing geriatric care through data science and intervention design. She is the author of Chapter 2.

Elizabeth H. Wheatley serves as Vice President of Resident Care at Benchmark Senior Living in Waltham, Massachusetts, USA. In this role, she provides strategic leadership and oversight for all aspects of resident care—including clinical services, social engagement, and memory care programming—across 70 assisted living communities throughout the Northeast. Prior to joining Benchmark, she spent nearly two decades with Five Star Senior Living, where she held senior leadership roles including Vice President of Health and Wellness and Corporate Director of Clinical Services. She is the co-author of Chapter 10.

Chapter 1
Assisted Living at the Crossroads

Helena Temkin-Greener and Sheryl Zimmerman

Introduction

Assisted living occupies a distinctive—and increasingly consequential—position in the U.S. long-term care landscape. Conceived as a middle ground between the medicalized environment of nursing homes and independent community living, the intent of assisted living has been to combine *assistance* with *living*: personal care and supportive services delivered in a residential setting that preserves dignity, autonomy, and individual choice. Embedded in this concept is a dual commitment—to provide care without trappings of "institutionalization" and support without undermining personhood. However, the care needs of assisted living residents have been evolving and so has the setting, as indicated by today's definition of assisted living [1]:

> Assisted living communities are licensed residential settings that provide housing; personal care; wellness, social, recreational, and health-related services, such as nursing and dementia care and 24-hour access to staff. These communities' core principles include person-centered services and policies, as well as an adequate number of well-trained, supported staff. Person-centered services and policies promote quality of life, privacy, choice, dignity, inclusion, and independence as defined by each individual and those who know them best.

More than three decades after its rapid expansion, scholars, policymakers, practitioners, residents, and families have come to ask a fundamental question: **is assisted living fulfilling its dual mission to provide assistance and support quality living?** [2]

H. Temkin-Greener (✉)
University of Rochester, Rochester, NY, USA
e-mail: Helena_Temkin-Greener@urmc.Rochester.edu

S. Zimmerman
University of North Carolina, Chapel Hill, NC, USA
e-mail: Sheryl_Zimmerman@unc.edu

H. Temkin-Greener and S. Zimmerman (eds.), *Assisted Living Through Research, Policy, and Practice*, https://doi.org/10.1007/978-3-032-32088-9_1

Growth in Assisted Living

For decades, assisted living has been the fastest-growing sector of residential long-term care in the U.S. From fewer than 100 communities in 1980, the sector has grown to more than 30,000 communities nationwide (Table 1.1). The scale and speed of this transformation are striking.

Between 1990 and 2000, while the number of nursing home beds increased by just 7 percent, residential care capacity, which included assisted living, grew by 97 percent [3].

Not surprisingly, assisted living expansion is tied to where the population of older adults has grown the fastest, meaning that states with rapidly increasing populations have seen greater demand and thus greater development. Today, California, followed by Florida, Arizona, Texas, and Wisconsin have the largest numbers of assisted living communities in the U.S. (Fig. 1.1), well in excess of 1500 each. And of course, as the number of assisted living communities increases so too does the total bed capacity. But, while states like California have the highest total number of beds, they tend to

Table 1.1 Evolution of assisted living communities in the U.S over Time

Decade / Year	Approximate Number of Assisted Living Communities	Notes / Source
1980	<100	Modern assisted living concept began in early 1980s
1990	No central data — *Emerging industry building out of historic residential care models*	Removal of nursing home-only dominance; assisted living expanding
1998	~11,500	National study estimated ~11,459 communities in 1998
2010	~36,000	According to 2009 HHS survey estimate
2020	~30,000+	Various reporting sources indicate more than 30,000 communities
2025	~30,500–32,000+	National Center for Assisted Living estimates ~32,231 communities with ~1.2 M beds.

Sources

U.S. Department of Health and Human Services, Administration on Aging, 2010. A profile of older Americans: 2010. Available at: https://acl.gov/sites/default/files/Aging%20and%20Disability%20in%20America/2010profile.pdf (Accessed: January 11, 2026).

National Academies of Sciences, Engineering, and Medicine. 2001. Improving the Quality of Long-Term Care. Washington, DC: The National Academies Press.

Hipp, D., 2024. Assisted living statistics and facts. Forbes. Available at: https://www.forbes.com/health/senior-living/assisted-living-statistics/ (Accessed: January 11, 2026).

American Health Care Association & National Center for Assisted Living (AHCA/NCAL), 2025. Assisted living facts and figures. Available at: https://www.ahcancal.org/Assisted-Living/Facts-and-Figures/Pages/default.aspx (Accessed: January 11, 2026).

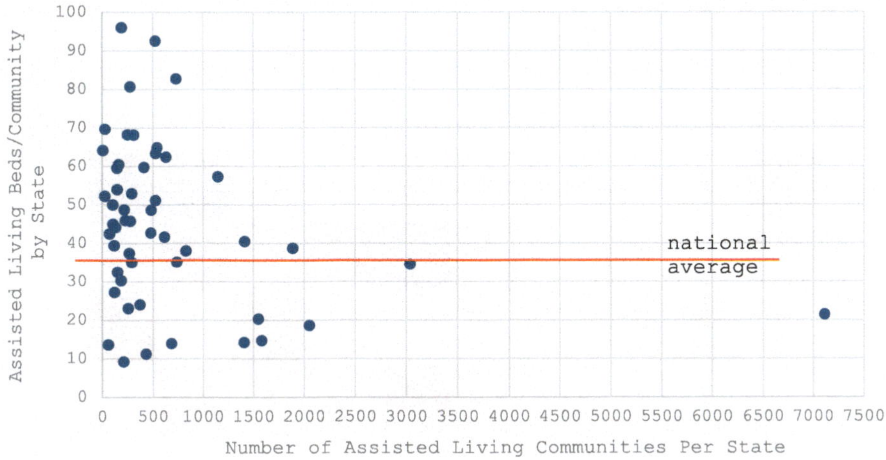

Fig. 1.1 Number of assisted living communities by average bed size: by State. *Source* Author's (HTG) database for 2019

have smaller communities with fewer beds in each (Fig. 1.2). California averages only 21.5 beds per community, suggesting a market dominated by smaller "board-and-care style" homes compared, for example, to Indiana's large-scale complexes with an average of almost 100 beds. In the Midwest and Northeast (Indiana, Ohio, New York, New Jersey) there is a considerable cluster of assisted living communities with the average bed size being significantly higher than the national average of 35 beds per community. Conversely, states like Alaska at 9.2 beds/community and Rhode Island at 13.7 beds tend to offer much smaller, likely more residential-style care models.

Expanding State Interest in Assisted Living

Over the past few decades, states' interest in assisted living as a means of reducing or delaying nursing home placement has significantly increased. State Medicaid long-term services and supports (LTSS) spending has shifted away from nursing homes toward home and community-based services (HCBS), which include services delivered in assisted living. Nationally, HCBS now constitutes the majority of Medicaid LTSS spending, and 41 state Medicaid programs cover some home care services for eligible assisted living residents [4]. Thirty four states cover personal care in assisted living and 29 make these services available around the clock. While these programs help assisted living residents who are Medicaid eligible to cover the cost of services, assisted living communities may not be eager to admit such residents as Medicaid payment rates are typically lower than private-pay rates. Today, only 10 states have policies that require assisted living communities to accept new residents who are enrolled in HCBS [4].

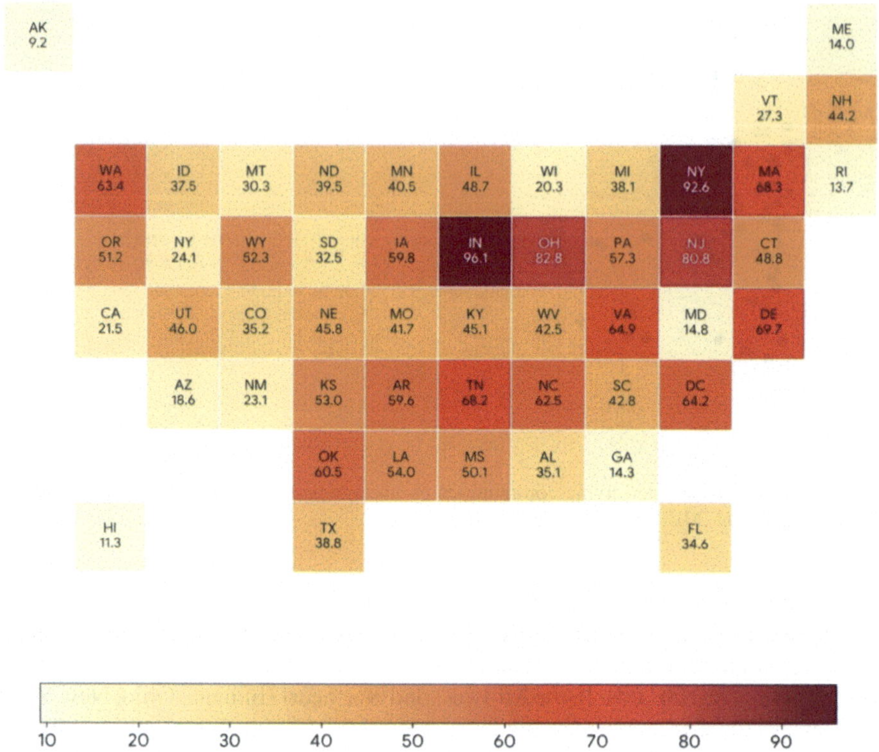

Fig. 1.2 Average number of beds per assisted living community: By state. *Source* Author's (HTG) database for 2019

Although most states cover some services in assisted living, many use waiver programs that have participant caps and waiting lists, meaning not all eligible people can access assisted living supports. Nationally, it is estimated that approximately 20% of assisted living residents rely on Medicaid [5], with significant variation by state; from virtually none in some states to more than 50% in a minority of others [6]. With increasing participation of Medicaid HCBS LTSS, assisted living has been pulled into the public safety net for older adults who need supportive care, creating new expectations around access, oversight, and quality—and perhaps even reshaping the financial pressures for the assisted living business model. On the one hand, Medicaid's growth in this sector expands the potential pool of residents by providing access to low and middle-income adults as they spend down their assets. On the other hand, many assisted living owners and providers may themselves cap the number of Medicaid residents they accept, or not accept any at all, because Medicaid service rates are lower than private-pay rates, and these residents tend to require more care than private-pay residents. This situation creates sharp market bifurcation with high-end, private-pay assisted living versus Medicaid-heavy communities that tend to be smaller with much thinner margins [7, 8].

Profitability as the Engine of Assisted Living Expansion

The growth of assisted living and other residential care settings in the last two decades reflects older adults' preferences for environments that emphasize person-centered care, autonomy, and the ability to age in place. Assisted living communities explicitly distinguished themselves from the historic "institutional" ethos of nursing home custodial care by marketing independence, privacy, dignity, and choice as defining features of the model [9, 10].

Assisted living expanded rapidly because its underlying business model combined housing and services in a way that was financially attractive to private payors and also to investors and operators. Unlike nursing homes, which are medical settings heavily reliant on Medicaid payment and subject to stringent federal rules, assisted living communities are licensed and regulated at the state level, and from a business perspective are structured as a hybrid real-estate plus service model. The hybrid model meant developers built communities for which residents paid monthly fees for private living spaces along with personal care and amenities—a model that generated robust gross profit margins often estimated between 25% and 35% for stabilized operations [11]. The assisted living industry has grown into a multibillion-dollar market, today valued at over $92 billion with projected strong growth reflecting demographic demand and investor interest. In this context, profitability was not an incidental outcome but a driver of expansion.

Changing Profitability and Resident Demographics Shaping the Assisted Living Model

As assisted living matured and states looked for lower-cost alternatives to nursing homes, Medicaid began to play a larger role in supporting services in assisted living settings. Medicaid enrollees who qualify for HCBS waivers or similar state plan options can now receive personal care services in assisted living if a community accepts Medicaid and has available rooms, although room and board usually are paid privately.

Research shows that states with more robust Medicaid financing options—including waivers and state plan coverage—have higher proportions of Medicaid and dual-eligible (i.e., Medicare and Medicaid) residents in assisted living than states without such coverage, evidencing that public payer policy influences both access and assisted living participation. This shift increases demand and occupancy but often narrows profit margins, because Medicaid reimbursement rates for HCBS services tend to be lower than private-pay rates and may not fully cover the cost of labor and care delivery. As operators consider accepting more Medicaid residents, they face a tradeoff: increased census and steady utilization versus thinner per-resident margins and greater administrative complexity.

The assisted living model is further evolving because the profile of residents and the cost structure of operations are changing simultaneously. Demographically, the population entering assisted living is older and has more complex care needs—including needing assistance with multiple activities of daily living and management of chronic conditions—compared to earlier cohorts. The industry as a whole serves a population predominantly older than age 80 with health needs that increasingly resemble people historically receiving care in nursing homes, but in a less clinical setting.

These demographic shifts carry implications for profitability. Care of higher-acuity residents requires more staff time and specialized training, and often raises labor costs—already the largest expense category for assisted living operations. At the same time, assisted living providers are responding with operational innovations and diversified revenue strategies—for example, tiered pricing for higher-level care, ancillary services, wellness programs, and technology adoption—to maintain financial viability.

This interplay of public payer shifts, resident acuity, and cost pressures have been pushing the sector toward hybrid care models that blend traditional assisted living with enhanced personal care and even medical care coordination. Such evolution reflects broader demographic and policy trends: an aging population requiring more support, shifts in long-term services and supports toward community settings, and a competitive landscape shaped by both public and private payment sources.

Why "Assisted Living Through Research, Policy, and Practice—What's in the Name?"

As the assisted living sector has evolved, research, practice, and policy have increasingly questioned whether assisted living does and can consistently deliver on its promises of "assistance" and "living." Residents now enter assisted living later in the aging trajectory, with greater functional impairment, medical complexity, and cognitive decline. Lengths of stay have shortened, workforce pressures have intensified, profit margins have shrunken, and regulatory oversight has become complex within and across states. Together, these trends have placed growing strain on a model originally designed for a healthier and more independent population, calling into question the alignment between assisted living's philosophical foundations and its contemporary realities [12].

This volume takes that tension—between *assistance* and *living*—as its point of departure. Bringing together leading scholars, clinicians, assisted living operators, residents, and consumer advocates, the chapters offer a comprehensive, research and practice-based examination of assisted living communities as they exist today. In so doing, they recognize both the promise and the challenge of assisted living noted in its definition: a setting that is residential rather than institutional, yet increasingly responsible for residents with complex and evolving care needs.

Readers will observe significant connecting threads within the chapters that follow. These threads reflect the lived reality of assisted living, where it is nearly impossible to examine any single aspect of residents' experiences in isolation. Regulation shapes workforce; workforce stability influences operators' ability to provide needed care; medical care provision and coordination, or the lack thereof, affect the use of health services such as hospitalizations and emergency care use, as well as dementia care, mental health, and end-of-life experiences; and all of these intersect with quality of life. Assisted living is not a modular system but an integrated social and care environment. The structure and contents of this volume mirror that interdependence.

Assisted Living in Context

As detailed by Wang in Chap. 2, *Assisted Living Communities and Their Residents*, today's assisted living residents are older and more medically complex than those of a generation ago. Many enter assisted living later in the aging process, often with multiple chronic conditions and cognitive impairment. As a result, the assisted living sector increasingly operates at the intersection of housing and health care—without necessarily being fully licensed as either. This positioning has profound implications. Communities must balance market appeal with their capacity to manage increasing levels of need. When residents' needs exceed a community's scope of care, transitions to hospitals, nursing homes, or hospice can be disruptive and distressing. These moments expose the complicated lines between assisted living's aspirational mission and its operational realities, underscoring the importance of transparency, coordination, and realistic expectations.

Regulation and the Boundaries of Care

As assisted living has expanded into a multibillion-dollar industry—encompassing both small, family-run homes and large corporate chains—its mission has become somewhat diffuse and diversity is the norm rather than the exception. This diversity is noted in state regulations that rely on 350 different licenses and certifications to govern assisted living [13]. Some states impose detailed staffing, training, and service requirements; others grant broad discretion to providers. While regulatory variability allows for flexibility as well as innovation, it also produces inconsistency and often inequity. Consumers may struggle to understand what services to expect, particularly across state lines, while providers face uneven oversight and accountability. As explored by Guo and Temkin-Greener in Chap. 3, *Assisted Living Regulations*, regulation does not merely set minimum standards; it actively shapes organizational behavior and defines the boundaries of responsibility—especially with respect to health-related services.

Workforce as the Foundation of Assistance

The capacity of assisted living communities to provide meaningful assistance and to promote living rests fundamentally on their workforce. Direct care workers—personal care aides, certified nursing assistants, and medication technicians—deliver most of the hands-on care and support. Yet, as examined by Schwartz in Chap. 4, *The Assisted Living Workforce*, these workers face chronic challenges, including low wages, limited benefits, high turnover, and constrained opportunities for advancement [14]. Workforce instability undermines continuity of care and weakens the relationships that are central to residents' sense of safety and well-being. It is particularly consequential for residents living with dementia, for whom consistent staffing is strongly associated with better quality of life [15]. Workforce challenges therefore cut across every domain of assisted living, shaping not only care delivery but also the feasibility of the sector's core mission.

The Expanse of Care Needs

In Chap. 5, Sloane, Zimmerman, Balter and Morton discuss *Dementia and Dementia Care in Assisted Living,* demonstrating the current centrality of dementia to the assisted living experience. A substantial proportion of residents live with Alzheimer's disease or related dementias, and many communities operate specialized memory care units. Supporting autonomy while ensuring safety, maintaining meaningful engagement, and navigating consent as cognition declines present ongoing ethical and practical challenges.

In addition, mental health concerns—including depression, anxiety, loneliness, and grief—are prevalent yet frequently underrecognized, as shown by Hua and Agundu in Chap. 6, *Mental Health Care in Assisted Living*. Residents may experience assisted living as both supportive and isolating: a place of safety that nevertheless does not maximize social connection and community engagement. Addressing mental health is therefore inseparable from promoting quality of life.

Although assisted living is not licensed as a medical setting, its residents increasingly require medical oversight, as clearly demonstrated by Howd and Caprio in Chap. 7, *Medical Care in Assisted Living*. Assisted living communities vary widely in how they respond to this reality. Some actively coordinate with physicians, nurse practitioners, home health agencies, and hospice providers; others focus more narrowly on assistance with activities of daily living. In some cases, families assume a level of clinical care that assisted living is neither required nor resourced to provide [16]; which can raise fundamental questions about accountability. Should assisted living revert to its original model of housing, or should it continue to evolve in response to the growing medical complexity of its residents? How these questions are answered will shape regulation, financing, workforce training, and the sector's future identity.

Finally, end-of-life care further underscores assisted living's evolving role, as described by Belanger in Chap. 8, *End-of-Life Care and Hospice.* Many residents wish to remain in place until death, and partnerships with hospice have expanded access to palliative care. At the same time, regulatory constraints, staffing limitations, and unclear clinical responsibility complicate this aspiration. Assisted living has thus become a site of dying as well as living, intensifying the stakes of how care is defined, delivered, and supported.

Defining and Measuring Quality

What constitutes quality in assisted living remains contested. Unlike nursing homes, assisted living lacks standardized national quality metrics. Regulators tend to emphasize safety and compliance, providers highlight amenities and lifestyle, families prioritize trust and responsiveness, and residents often define quality in terms of autonomy, relationships, and a sense of home. This volume, as detailed by Kemp in Chap. 9 *Quality of Care and Quality of Life*, adopts a holistic conception of quality that integrates care outcomes with quality of life.

Perspectives of Providers and Consumers

The focus of this volume is on the research evidence about the extent to which assisted living communities are meeting their original intent of "assisted" and "living." Nevertheless, such a volume would not be complete without including the perspectives of both providers and consumers (consumer advocates). These are explored in Chap. 10, *Perspectives of Providers and Consumer Advocates Regarding 'Assisted' and 'Living'*. This chapter is fundamental and intentionally different from those preceding it. Through discussion groups with assisted living providers and consumer advocates, Moczygemba and colleagues present the perspectives of these participants on the eight core themes explored in this volume. The groups shared many similar perspectives and acknowledged challenges related to assisted living affordability and workforce, but providers seemed more optimistic emphasizing innovation and successes vis-à-vis person-centered care, while consumers were more likely to express concern about the extent to which residents and their families clearly understood, upon admission, assisted living limitations vis-à-vis services and care provision, and were more hesitant about residents' rights protections. Both groups had recommendations related to the promise of "assisted" and "living," and noted that other solutions are "still waiting to be discovered."

Conclusion

Assisted Living in Transition and at a Policy Juncture

Assisted living is in transition and at a policy juncture. It has moved from the margins to the center of aging and long-term care policy in the U.S. It now serves a population that is older, frailer, and more medically complex than originally envisioned, while operating within regulatory and financing frameworks that differ within and across states. As a result, assisted living occupies an evolving position: expected to support aging in place and accommodate increasing care needs, yet needing practice, policy, and reimbursement that meet those expectations.

The central question animating this volume—whether assisted living fulfills its promise of providing both "*assistance*" and "*living*" - is therefore not merely conceptual. It is fundamentally empirical and relevant to practice and policy. Decisions about licensure, staffing requirements, scope of practice, Medicaid coverage, quality oversight, and integration with health care systems all shape what assisted living should and can realistically deliver, and for whom. The absence of a coherent national framework has enabled flexibility and innovation, but it has also produced wide variations in access, quality, and accountability.

Taken together, the chapters in this volume demonstrate that "*assistance*" and "*living*" are not competing goals but interdependent dimensions of quality. Preserving both requires intentional alignment across regulation, financing, workforce, and organizational practice. Policies or practices that privilege one at the expense of the other risk eroding the very grounding of assisted living.

Implications for "Assistance" and "Living"

At the heart of assisted living is the balance it seeks to strike between *assistance* and *living*. The evidence presented in this volume suggests that maintaining this balance has become increasingly complex as resident acuity rises and expectations for care expand. The challenge is not simply whether assisted living provides sufficient assistance, but whether assistance is delivered in ways that truly promote quality of life. In parallel, the nursing home industry has been undergoing its own transformation coined "culture change" more than 15 years ago. This movement has been working to transition nursing homes to a more home-like environment, with the key elements being person-centered care, staff empowerment, a more home-like environment, close relationships between residents/families and staff, and continuous quality improvement [17]; an uncanny resemblance to the assisted living playbook as nursing homes have sought to shake their "institutional" persona.

Assistance in assisted living extends beyond task completion or clinical oversight. It includes relational continuity, responsiveness to changing needs of the residents, and the capacity to provide support without eroding autonomy. When staffing is unstable, training inadequate, or clinical responsibility unclear, assistance may become fragmented or reactive, undermining both safety and quality of life.

At the same time, *living* in assisted living communities entails more than residential amenities or physical design. Living encompasses autonomy, privacy, meaningful activity, social connection, and a sense of home. These dimensions are often most vulnerable when care needs intensify, when risk management supersedes resident preferences, or when regulatory and liability concerns constrain everyday life.

Implications for Research

The chapters in this volume point to several priorities for future research. First, there is a need for longitudinal, resident-centered studies that track health, function, cognition, quality of life, and care transitions over time. Much of the existing evidence relies on cross-sectional designs or community-level data, limiting understanding of how well assisted living supports residents as needs evolve.

Second, the lack of standardized national quality measures underscores the importance of developing valid and comparable indicators that reflect both care outcomes and lived experience. Research must extend beyond compliance-based metrics to capture autonomy, dignity, social engagement, and person-centered care—core dimensions of assisted living that are difficult to measure but central to its mission. Mixed-methods approaches that integrate administrative and claims data, resident and family perspectives, and observational research may be particularly well suited to this task.

Third, the pronounced variation in state regulation presents an opportunity for policy-relevant research. Differences in licensure standards, Medicaid waiver design, staffing requirements, and scope of practice function as natural experiments, allowing examination of how policy choices shape access, quality, workforce stability, and resident outcomes. Comparative analyses across states—and, where possible, internationally—can help identify policy configurations that better align assisted living's aspirations with its operational realities.

Finally, future research must more fully engage with the assisted living workforce. Understanding recruitment, retention, training, job quality, and career pathways is essential to assessing both quality and sustainability. Without a stable, supported workforce, the promise of assisted living cannot be realized, regardless of regulatory intent or organizational mission.

Implications for Policy

The findings in this volume suggest that future policy debates should move beyond binary distinctions—housing versus health care, social versus medical models—and instead recognize assisted living as an inherently hybrid setting. Policies that fail to acknowledge this hybridity risk either overmedicalizing a residential environment or under-supporting residents with substantial and increasing needs.

Several policy implications emerge. First, regulatory frameworks must more clearly define expectations for care while preserving flexibility for person-centered practice. This change includes greater clarity regarding scope of services, staffing competencies, and accountability for health-related care, particularly for residents with dementia and other complex conditions.

Second, financing mechanisms—especially Medicaid waivers—must be better aligned with the level and intensity of services that assisted living residents require. As public financing expands, so too does the need for transparency and accountability regarding quality, access, and equity.

Third, workforce policy is central. Investments in training, compensation, and career advancement are not ancillary concerns but foundational to quality and sustainability. Without addressing workforce instability, regulatory and financing reforms are unlikely to achieve their intended effects.

Finally, policy approaches must recognize assisted living as an increasingly important site of end-of-life care. Supporting residents' preferences to remain in place will require clearer integration with hospice and palliative care, as well as regulatory and reimbursement policies that support, rather than impede, these partnerships.

Closing Comment

Assisted living will continue to play a critical role in long-term care across the US, whether by design or by default. The question is not whether the sector will expand, but under what conditions and with what expectations. By examining the gap between promise and practice, and by integrating perspectives from residents, families, providers, and policymakers, this volume provides a foundation for more informed research, more coherent policy, and more intentional practice—aimed at ensuring that assisted living can more fully realize its commitment to both *assistance* and *living* in the years ahead.

Competing Interests The authors have no conflicts of interest to declare that are relevant to the content of this chapter.

References

1. Zimmerman, S. Toward a common definition of assisted living. September 2024. Available at https://www.mcknightsseniorliving.com/home/columns/guest-columns/toward-a-common-definition-of-assisted-living/.
2. Zimmerman S, Stone RI, Carder P, Thomas K. Does assisted living provide assistance and promote living? Health Aff. 2024;43:674–81.

3. Harrington C, Chapman S, Newcomer R. Trends in the supply of long-term-care facilities and beds in the United States. Journal of Appplied Gerontology. 2005;24:265–80.
4. Chidambaram P, Wolk A, Burns A, Watts M. What Services Does Medicaid Cover in Assisted Living Facilities? Haiser Family Foundation2025.
5. Temkin-Greener H, Mao Y, McGarry B, Li Y, et al. Using Medicare enrollment Data Base to identify beneficiaries in assisted living. JAMDA. 2022;
6. Hipp D. Assisted living statistics and facts. Forbes. 2024; Available at: https://www.forbes.com/health/senior-living/assisted-living-statistics/ (Accessed: January 11, 2026)
7. Cornell PY, Hua C, Rahman M, et al. Association of Medicaid Financing and Concentration of assisted living residents dually eligible for Medicare and Medicaid. JAMA Health Forum. 2023;4:e225338.
8. Gunderson R, Smith L, Cornell PY, Carder P, Thomas K. Medicaid mechanisms and state licensure: pathways to payment in assisted living. JAMDA. 2026;27:1–4.
9. Kane RL, Cutler DM. Re-imagining long-term services and supports: toward livable environments, service capacity, and community integration. Gerontologist. 2009;49:286–95.
10. Chapin RK. Home and community-based services: assuring quality in long-term care. J Aging and Social Policy. 2001;12:1–22.
11. Assisted Living Undustry. Statistics. 2026; (Accessed January 15, 2026, at https://gitnux.org/assisted-living-industry-statistics/?utm_source=chatgpt.com
12. Zimmerman S, Carder P, Schwartz L, et al. The imperative to reimagine assisted living. J Am Med Dir Assoc. 2022;23:225–34.
13. Smith L, Carder P, Bucy T, et al. Connecting policy to licensed assisted living communities, introducing health services regulatory analysis. Health Serv Res. 2021;56:540–9.
14. Stone RI, Bryant NS. The future of the home care workforce: training, supports, and job quality. Gerontologist. 2019;59:e294–303.
15. Zimmerman S, Cohen LW, Washington T, Ward K, Giorgio P. Evaluating measures and instruments for quality improvement in assisted living | managed health care connect. Annals of Long-Term Care: Clinical Care and Aging; 2016.
16. Ball MM, Perkins MM, Whittington FJ, et al. Managing decline in assisted living: the key to aging in place. J Gerontol B Psychol Sci Soc Sci. 2004;59B:S202–S12.
17. Koren MJ. Person-Centered Care for Nursing Home Residents:The Culture-Change Movement. Health Aff 2010;29.

Chapter 2
Assisted Living Communities and their Residents

Jinjiao Wang

Introduction

Assisted living communities are the fastest-growing sector in the residential long-term care industry in the United States [1–5]. Today, assisted living is the largest long-term care provider, with approximately 32,200 communities offering 1.2 million residential care beds [2, 4]. Over the years, the assisted living model has transformed from primarily offering hospitality, providing room and board along with basic personal and supportive services, into a hybrid model with different levels of care serving residents with increasingly complex clinical care needs [1, 7, 8]. Approximately 64% of residents require assistance with bathing, 50% with walking and dressing, 38% with toileting, and 30% with bed transfers, highlighting the high acuity in many communities [4].

Services Provided in Assisted Living Communities

Assisted living communities offer 24-hour supervision, wellness and social programs, medication assistance (depending on state regulations), transportation, and assistance with activities of daily living. The vast majority (81.9%) of communities are for-profit, with 56% belonging to chains and 42% independently owned. Assisted living communities vary widely with regard to bed capacity, with approximately 46% having four to 10 beds, 15% having 11 to 25 beds, 32% having 26 to 100 beds, and 8% having more than 100 beds; the average bed count is 37 licensed beds [9, 10]. Importantly, although assisted living residents often live with multiple

J. Wang (✉)
University of Texas at San Antonio Health Science Center, San Antonio, TX, USA
e-mail: wangj17@uthscsa.edu

H. Temkin-Greener and S. Zimmerman (eds.), *Assisted Living Through Research, Policy, and Practice*, https://doi.org/10.1007/978-3-032-32088-9_2

medical conditions, continued skilled nursing care is not routinely provided in this care setting, unlike in nursing homes.

As noted in a recently published commentary, the assisted living concept has evolved over time, offering a variety of models and services, while highlighting its premise to provide person-centered services ("assistance") designed to minimize the need to move ("living") [11].

Since its inception, assisted living has been an evolving concept, one that is shaped more by local experimentation than by a national design [11]. Early models featuring board-and-care homes offered little more than room and board, but by the late 1980s and early 1990s, new models began to emerge. Among these new models, some, like Oregon's approach, emphasized resident autonomy and provided health-related services. Others, e.g., those in the East Coast, focused more on hospitality and supportive amenities. Today, assisted living communities still vary broadly in the services they offer, staffing levels and ratios, and philosophies, particularly in balancing the promise between "assistance" and "living." Some emphasize apartment-style units and communal dining with personal and supportive services available a la carte. Others include some personal care and limited clinical oversight in their base price with additional services available for purchase as needed. Though such variations may reflect flexibility for both the residents and the providers, they beg a deeper question: what does it really mean to be "assisted" and to be "living" in these settings? As residents' needs grow more complex, the tensions between the support provided ("assisted") and the quality of life ("living") become harder to ignore and more urgent to address [11].

State Variations in Assisted Living Presence

Assisted living market penetration parallels the population's care needs as the number of individuals who may need such services varies geographically. States with large, older adult populations (e.g., California, Florida, Texas, Michigan) have the largest number of assisted living communities, whereas their presence is sparser in states with smaller populations (e.g., Hawaii, Wyoming, Delaware). In general, Western regional dominance of assisted living industry is not coincidental, but underscores population growth of older adults and market conditions that support investment in residential care infrastructure (e.g., higher incomes, preference for independent living) that fuel both the supply of and the demand for assisted living communities in these regions [4, 12].

Beyond geographic distribution, considerable state-level variation exists in the terms used to describe assisted living communities. States use a large array of names for communities that provide housing, supportive services, and personal care assistance to older adults, including "assisted living" (the one used here), "residential care facilities," "residential care homes," "personal care homes," "board and care homes," "rest homes," "adult care homes," and "supported living," among others. This array of terminology not only reflects the evolving nature of such residential care settings, but perhaps more so variations in state-based regulatory approaches to assisted living communities. In contrast to nursing home regulations, which are largely based on national standards, assisted living communities are predominantly state regulated and these regulations can be very different from one state to another. Such variance underscores the complexity of the assisted living landscape, results in broad variability in oversight and services, as well as safety standards [7–9, 13–15].

Cost and Financing of Assisted Living Services

In 2024 the annual median cost for assisted living stay was $70,800 or $5900 monthly [6], which is significantly higher than the median annual household income of adults aged 65 and older (i.e., $52,290 according to the U.S. Census Bureau, 2023 data) [16]. Most assisted living residents are Medicare beneficiaries, but the services provided by these communities are primarily financed through private pay using personal savings, pensions, or retirement income [16]. A small proportion of residents supplement these costs with private long-term care insurance, although coverage and limits vary by policy [17]. For those who are dually eligible for Medicare and Medicaid, Medicaid may cover the cost of some personal care, but not room and board, through Home- and Community-Based Services (HCBS) waivers or managed care programs. The eligibility for and availability of HCBS differ widely across states, and not all assisted living communities accept Medicaid rates [18]. Additionally, veterans may access aid through the Veterans Affairs' Aid and Attendance Pension Benefit to help cover costs [19, 20]. Overall, financing of services in assisted living often involves a mix of these sources tailored to the residents' financial situation, state-specific programs, and each community's willingness to work with them.

Dually Eligible Beneficiaries in Assisted Living

In 2024, approximately 12.8 million individuals were dually eligible for Medicare and Medicaid [21], representing about 20% of Medicare enrollees [22, 23]. While dually eligible beneficiaries are less likely to reside in assisted living than those who are Medicare-only, they make up a significant and growing portion of this population. Nearly one in five (18%) of assisted living residents have their care paid partially through Medicaid [24]. Because Medicaid programs are regulated at the state levels, there are differences in how services in assisted living communities are covered across states. Therefore, the scope of coverage available to Medicaid beneficiaries in assisted living varies depending on the specific policies of each state. Some states allow such services under HCBS waivers or managed care contracts, while others do not [18]. As of 2024, 41 states and the District of Columbia offer Medicaid-funded HCBS in assisted living communities, mainly through 1915(c) waivers or managed care contracts, whereas services in other states are not provided or are very limited [25, 26]. For example, Texas offers limited HCBS under its Medicaid program and may not cover all assisted living services [27]. Access to assisted living for the dually eligible beneficiaries is also limited by state-imposed waiting lists and funding availability [18, 28].

Assisted Living Residents

Resident Characteristics

Nationally, at least half of assisted living residents are aged 85 and older and most have co-morbid chronic conditions. Over 40% have Alzheimer's disease or other dementias, 38% have heart disease, more than 60% have arthritis, and almost 40% have diabetes [29]. Functional impairments are also widespread, as mentioned earlier.

Serious mental illness is also prominent though variability exists in the exact prevalence. Overall, more than 50% of the residents have a diagnosis of major depression, almost 16% have schizophrenia, and 12% bipolar disorder [30]. Chronic pain is significant, affecting approximately 20% of the residents [31, 32].

Similar to other older Americans, assisted living residents face polypharmacy: taking five or more medications is common in this population, with over half (51%) taking six or more medications daily [33]. Potentially inappropriate medications, that is, medications that may cause the resident more harm than benefit, and medications that are likely no longer necessary given changes in a resident's health status, are also common in this population. For example, at least one fifth of assisted living residents are found to take antipsychotics regularly [34], even though this medication class is associated with increased risk of mortality when used among individuals with dementia [30–38], suggesting a need for a comprehensive, patient-centered medication review, which does not frequently happen even in well-managed medical care settings.

In sum, assisted living residents present a high prevalence of chronic disease, cognitive impairment, complex medication regimens, and functional limitations, underscoring the need for comprehensive care strategies that address medical, cognitive, and daily-living supports [10, 14, 31, 32, 39–43].

Assisted Living Residents Versus Community-Dwelling Older Adults

Assisted living residents generally are older and have greater health and functional needs as well as worse health outcomes (e.g., falls, death, hospitalization, emergency room visits) than community-dwelling older adults [44–48]. Assisted living communities often provide specialized dementia care or memory support services, which are not typically available in the community setting. In contrast, community-dwelling older adults may need to rely on family and community networks for dementia services and support. Theoretically, due to the structure of assisted living communities (e.g., group housing and organized activities in shared space), compared to living in one's own home, assisted living offers a built-in social environment with opportunities for community engagement, structured activities, and peer interaction. However, existing studies have suggested that though assisted living is a setting with great promise to engage residents to be more active and socially connected [49], many residents do experience loneliness, depression and inactivity as well as social isolation [50]. This may stem from feelings and perceptions of abandonment and not being needed and wanted by their families, as well as due to rules and regulations that erode personal freedom and privacy, ultimately weakening individuals' sense of social identity and self-worth [51]. Many assisted living residents express a desire for more meaningful activities and nature-based experiences [52, 53].

Assisted living residents may benefit from having staff available to assist with activities of daily living, monitor health status, and respond to emergencies; however, the extent and quality of this support varies considerably across communities, particularly as many do not provide on-site medical care and residents rely on external healthcare providers similar to community-dwelling older adults [8, 17]. Assisted living communities may also benefit by improving safety culture and incorporating more safety features such as emergency response systems, fall prevention measures, and structured routines that may reduce certain risks (e.g., medication errors, delayed response to acute events) [15, 54], as compared to older adults managing these tasks independently at home with or without caregiver support. Community-dwelling older adults without strong in-home support may face greater challenges in coordinating care, managing medications safely, and responding promptly to health emergencies, though access to home health services [55], telehealth [56], and strong social networks [57] can mitigate some of these risks. In assisted living, the protective value of safety features depends heavily on staff availability, training adequacy, and regulatory oversight, which vary markedly by state and across communities [58].

Assisted Living Residents Versus Nursing Home Residents

Historically, assisted living communities have served predominantly older adults with moderate care needs who prefer a residential, homelike environment, while nursing homes have provided care for individuals with higher acuity requiring skilled nursing services. As a result, assisted living residents are generally expected to be less medically complex and more functionally independent than nursing home residents. However, over the past three decades, this distinction has blurred considerably. Research shows that increasing numbers of assisted living residents exhibit complex medical conditions, cognitive impairment, and higher care needs that traditionally have been expected of nursing home residents [2, 59–61], but these findings are not unequivocal. For example, it has been shown that the medical acuity and complexity of nursing home residents remains higher than that of assisted living residents [24], and that factors influencing one's admission to assisted living or nursing home often extend beyond care needs and include socioeconomic status, availability of support at home and individual/family preferences [60, 61].

Decision Making Regarding Assisted Living Transitions

Key Factors Influencing Admission to Assisted Living

Given that traditional housing is still the most preferred residential option among older adults [62], admissions to assisted living are often driven by need—that is, increase in care needs that are not being met at home. Placement decisions reflect a mix of health needs, social support, finances, and available services. This is reflected by studies finding that compared to older adults who continue to live in traditional community housing, new assisted living residents are more likely to be cognitively impaired [63], have complex health conditions including medical diagnoses and mental health concerns, have overall higher care needs, and are more likely to be without a partner as their primary caregiver, thus without adequate support at home [64]. In general, several factors have been found to influence older adults' decision for assisted living admission: health status, financial status, availability of home support, and assisted living availability.

Health Status. Chronic conditions such as dementia, cognitive impairment, and functional decline in activities of daily living (ADLs) and instrumental activities (IADLs) are strong predictors of assisted living admission decisions [63, 65]. Recent hospitalizations or acute health events can also precipitate the move to assisted living, likely due to heightened functional decline surrounding hospitalization and family's greater awareness of older adults' complex care needs that typically follow a hospital discharge [24, 63, 66].

Socioeconomic Considerations and Support at Home. Since assisted living stays are mostly privately funded, as stated previously, affordability plays a significant role [63, 67]. Preferences for level of care versus cost, personal preference for autonomy, and quality of life in different settings are weighed in one's (and/or their family) decision to enter assisted living versus alternative care settings, including nursing homes [68, 69]. Availability and capacity of informal caregivers such as spouses or adult children, as well as availability of additional, paid caregiver support is likely to influence timing and likelihood of assisted living admission [69, 70]. Living arrangements (alone or with others) and caregiver burnout also impact these decisions, especially when the older adult has chronic conditions that substantially compound their care needs, such as dementia [71, 72]. Community-dwelling older adults who initially received more visits from home-visiting professionals, such as physical therapists and aides, were also found to transition to assisted living at a later time [73].

Availability of Assisted Living Beds. Geographic access, waiting lists, and specialized service availability (e.g., memory care for those living with dementia) also impact assisted living admission [4, 8]. Characteristics of communities such as profit status and staffing levels may affect their capacity to admit individuals with greater care needs. For example, assisted living communities with above-average personal care staffing levels, and the for-profit communities, are more likely to admit residents who need assistance with feeding and bathing, and less likely to discharge or transition them to a higher level of care setting such as nursing homes [74].

How to Prepare for Assisted Living Admission?

Though assisted living admissions are mostly driven by ongoing care needs [75], many new residents may find this a difficult transition to deal with, as described in existing qualitative studies. New residents shared feelings of loss of autonomy and independence, downsizing to space that results in loss of belongings, emotional distress, social disconnection, and even cultural dissonance, thus emphasizing the need for pre-admission planning and culturally sensitive care in assisted living communities [76–78]. These findings urge more research to examine how residents can be better supported through community- and assisted living-based programs before, during and after the decision to enter these communities. Prior studies have identified strategies that can help older adults ease into the new assisted living environment, for example through focusing on relationship-centered care and connectedness—ensuring continuity of care, homelike environment with personal belongings and decorations, and culturally sensitive caring practices, including diet, language, and social activities [79, 80].

Reasons for Leaving Assisted Living

The average length of stay in assisted living is 22 months ranging from 1 to 3 years, with considerable variability. Assisted living residents may leave due to transitions to nursing homes, which happen in 60% of the cases, hospitalizations, or death [81]. Research has shown that at 12 months more than one fourth of the residents have relocated or died [81].

Transitions from assisted living communities to nursing homes are often driven by declining health, including urinary incontinence, functional impairment, depression, cognitive decline, and insufficient access to on-site medical or skilled nursing services [81–84]. An eight-year longitudinal study identified poorer physical performance and lower educational attainment (less than a college degree) as significant predictors of nursing home placement among assisted living residents, whereas those who remained physically active were markedly less likely to experience such transitions [85]. Importantly, as residents' health deteriorates, some communities support the use of home-based clinical services—such as visiting nurses and home health care providers—to help bridge care gaps and delay nursing home admission when assisted living resources are limited [86]. Additionally, Medicare-Medicaid dually eligible beneficiaries have been shown to experience higher hospitalization rates and higher rates of transitions to custodial nursing home care compared to the Medicare-only assisted living residents, highlighting the compounded vulnerability of this population [87, 88].

To reduce the residents' risk of transitions such as hospitalization or nursing home placement, it is key that assisted living be properly and adequately staffed. For example, higher registered nurse staffing levels in assisted living are associated with lower risk of injuries and hospitalizations among the residents, particularly those with dementia [89, 90].

Perhaps due to the buffering effects of services provided in assisted living, the residents who have comparable health profiles to community-dwelling older adults are less likely to transition to nursing homes than their community-dwelling counterparts [91]. Given that some assisted living communities permit admission and retention of residents with nursing home–level care needs, it is critical that communities conduct accurate admission assessments and ongoing reassessments to monitor residents' evolving needs, ensure adequate service delivery, and facilitate timely transfers to higher levels of care when appropriate [75].

Implications for "Assisted" and "Living"

Many assisted living communities remain insufficiently staffed to meet the complex medical and cognitive needs of today's resident population. Key challenges include continued reliance on off-site medical providers; memory care units that are often siloed, understaffed, or underperforming; inadequate staff-to-resident ratios; and a workforce frequently lacking the specialized training necessary to manage geriatric multimorbidity, neurocognitive disorders, and chronic disease management [42]. These systemic shortcomings have contributed to unmet needs among assisted living residents and underscore the growing tensions between the assisted living intent to serve as a primarily non-medical, residential care model and the heightened acuity of the population it now serves [3, 11].

As assisted living communities are increasingly called upon to accommodate residents with more medically acute care needs, many have recognized that this shift requires navigating a delicate, and at times conflicting, balance between preserving the core principles of autonomy, independence, and residential character, while simultaneously ensuring safety and compliance with regulatory and legal standards [92–94].

This evolving landscape presents not only operational challenges but also raises critical safety, ethical, and legal concerns. As highlighted by the American College of Physicians [92], the traditional autonomy-centered promise of assisted living communities must now be reconciled with the real-world care demands of increasingly frail, medically vulnerable populations. Notably, evidence from the COVID-19 pandemic, in Alberta, Canada, revealed that the rate of excess mortality among assisted living residents exceeded that of nursing home residents [95], underscoring the potential dangers associated with housing high-acuity individuals in settings that may lack the infrastructure, staffing, or clinical resources to respond to public health crises, or to provide routine medical care needs.

In conclusion, the evolving assisted living landscape characterized by high and increasing resident acuity, complex health profiles, and a growing proportion of dually eligible Medicare-Medicaid beneficiaries, poses substantial challenges to the founding vision of assisted living model as a supportive, non-institutional and non-medical setting that balances assistance with independence. While assisted living communities continue to deliver vital personal care and supportive services, the rising clinical complexity of their residents often places considerable strain on staff, resources, and the social fabric of these communities. This, in turn, may compromise some residents' ability to obtain enough "assistance" to continue "living" in their community safely with autonomy, purposeful engagement, and sustained quality of life. To honor the dual promise of 'assisted' and 'living,' these communities must continue to evolve, perhaps embracing integrated care models, investing in staff education and interdisciplinary training, and embedding person-centered practices that uphold dignity while meeting the increasingly intricate needs of the residents they serve.

Competing Interests The author has no conflicts of interest to declare that are relevant to the content of this chapter.

References

1. Zimmerman S, Gruber-Baldini AL, Sloane PD, et al. Assisted living and nursing homes: apples and oranges? The Gerontologist. 2003;43(suppl_2):107-117
2. Grabowski DC, Stevenson DG, Cornell PY. Assisted living expansion and the market for nursing home care. Health Serv Res. 2012;47(6):2296–315. https://doi.org/10.1111/j.1475-6773.2012.01425.x.
3. Zimmerman S, Carder P, Schwartz L, et al. The imperative to reimagine assisted living. J Am Med Dir Assoc. 2022;23(2):225–34. https://doi.org/10.1016/j.jamda.2021.12.004.
4. Grand View Research. *U.S. Assisted Living Facility Market Size,* Share & trends analysis report by age (more than 85, 75–84, 65–74, less than 65), *Region (West,* South, Midwest), And Segment Forecasts, *2022–2030.* 2022. Accessed November 1, 2022. https://www.grandviewresearch.com/industry-analysis/us-assisted-living-facility-market#:~:text=The%20U.S.%20assisted%20living%20facility,5.48%25%20from%202022%20to%202030.
5. U.S. Department of Health and Human Services CfDCaP, National Center for Health Statistics. *Post-acute and Long-term Care Providers and Services Users in the United States, 2017–2018: Analytical and Epidemiological Studies.* 2022. *Vital and Health Statistics Centers.* Accessed November 1, 2022. https://www.cdc.gov/nchs/data/series/sr_03/sr03-047.pdf
6. Genworth. Cost of Care Survey Tool. 2024. Accessed, November 12, 2025. https://seniornavigator.org/article/97426/genworth-cost-care-survey-tool

7. Thomas KS, Zhang W, Cornell PY, Smith L, Kaskie B, Carder PC. State variability in the prevalence and healthcare utilization of assisted living residents with dementia. J Am Geriatr Soc. 2020;68(7):1504–11. https://doi.org/10.1111/jgs.16410.
8. Han K, Trinkoff AM, Storr CL, Lerner N, Yang BK. Variation across U.S. assisted living facilities: admissions, resident care needs, and staffing. J Nurs Scholarsh. 2017;49(1):24–32. https://doi.org/10.1111/jnu.12262.
9. Caffrey C, Sengupta M. Variation in residential care community resident characteristics, by size of community: United States, 2016. NCHS Data Brief. 2018;299:1–8.
10. Long-term Care Providers and Services Users in the United States, 2015–2016. (2019).
11. Zimmerman S, Stone R, Carder P, Thomas K. Does assisted living provide assistance and promote living? Health Aff (Millwood). 2024;43(5):674–81. https://doi.org/10.1377/hlthaff.2023.00972.
12. Miller KEM, Zhao J, Laine LT, Coe NB. Growth of private pay senior housing communities in metropolitan statistical areas in the United States: 2015-2019. Med Care Res Rev. 2023;80(1):101–8. https://doi.org/10.1177/10775587221106121.
13. Temkin-Greener H, Mao Y, Ladwig S, Cai X, Zimmerman S, Li Y. Variability and potential determinants of assisted living state regulatory stringency. J Am Med Dir Assoc. 2021;22(8):1714–1719.e2. https://doi.org/10.1016/j.jamda.2020.10.014.
14. Rome V, Harris-Kojetin L, Carder P. Variation in licensed nurse staffing characteristics by state requirements in residential care. Res Gerontol Nurs. 2019;12(1):27–33. https://doi.org/10.3928/19404921-20181212-03.
15. Temkin-Greener H, Mao Y, McGarry B, Zimmerman S. Patient safety culture in assisted living: staff perceptions and association with state regulations. J Am Med Dir Assoc Dec 2022;23(12):1997–2002.e3. doi:https://doi.org/10.1016/j.jamda.2022.09.007.
16. United States Census Bureau. Income in the United States: 2023. Updated August. 2024;30. Accessed June 26, 2025, https://www.census.gov/library/publications/2024/demo/p60-282.html
17. Kisling-Rundgren A, Paul DP. 3rd, Coustasse a. costs, staffing, and Services of Assisted Living in the United States: a literature review. Health Care Manag (Frederick) Apr-Jun. 2016;35(2):156–63. https://doi.org/10.1097/hcm.0000000000000107.
18. Fabius CD, Cornell PY, Zhang W, Thomas KS. State Medicaid Financing and Access to Large Assisted Living Settings for Medicare–Medicaid Dual-Eligibles. Med Care Res Rev 2022;79(1):69–77. doi:https://doi.org/10.1177/1077558720987666.
19. U.S. Department of Veterans Affairs. VA aid and attendance benefits and housebound allowance. Update. 2024; Accessed July 2, 2025, https://www.va.gov/pension/aid-attendance-housebound/
20. U.S. Department of Veterans Affairs. VA Benefits for Elderly Veterans. Updated June 21, 2025. Accessed July 2, 2025, https://www.benefits.va.gov/persona/veteran-elderly.asp
21. The Commonwealth Fund. The Health Care Experiences of People Dually Eligible for Medicare and Medicaid. Updated June 27, 2024. Accessed June 26, 2025, https://www.commonwealthfund.org/publications/2024/jun/health-care-experiences-people-dually-eligible-medicare-medicaid#:~:text=People%20enrolled%20in%20both%20Medicare,and%20those%20in%20traditional%20Medicare.
22. The Kaiser Family Foundation. A profile of Medicare-Medicaid enrollees (dual eligibles). Updated January. 2023;31. https://www.kff.org/medicare/issue-brief/a-profile-of-medicare-medicaid-enrollees-dual-eligibles/
23. Medicare payment advisory commission and the Medicaid and CHIP payment and access commission. Data Book: Beneficiaries Dually Eligible for Medicare and Medicaid 2024. https://www.macpac.gov/wp-content/uploads/2024/01/Jan24_MedPAC_MACPAC_DualsDataBook-508.pdf
24. Wang J, Mao Y, McGarry B, Cai S, Temkin-Greener H. Assisted living or nursing home: who is moving in? J Am Geriatr Soc Nov 2023;71(11):3480–3488. doi:https://doi.org/10.1111/jgs.18503.

25. Medicaid.gov. Home & Community-Based Services 1915(c). Accessed July 2, 2025, https://www.medicaid.gov/medicaid/home-community-based-services/home-community-based-services-authorities/home-community-based-services-1915c
26. Watts MO, Musumeci M, Ammula M. State policy choices about Medicaid home and community-based services amid the pandemic (issue brief). Kaiser Family Foundation. 2022;
27. National Council on Aging. Assisted Living in Texas. Updated Oct 3, 2024. Accessed July 2, 2025, https://www.ncoa.org/adviser/local-care/assisted-living/texas/
28. Medicaid Assisted Living Services: Improved Federal Oversight of beneficiary health and welfare is needed (2018).
29. Zimmerman S, Guo W, Mao Y, Li Y, Temkin-Greener H. Health care needs in assisted living: survey data may underestimate chronic conditions. J Am Med Dir Assoc. 2021;22(2):471–3.
30. Temkin-Greener H, Guo W, McGarry B, Cai S. Serious mental illness in assisted living communities: association with nursing home placement. J Am Med Dir Assoc. 2024;25(5):917–22. https://doi.org/10.1016/j.jamda.2024.02.015.
31. Resnick B, Boltz M, Galik E, et al. Pain assessment, management, and impact among older adults in assisted living. Pain Manag Nurs. 2019;20(3):192–7. https://doi.org/10.1016/j.pmn.2019.02.008.
32. Zimmerman S, Sloane PD, Reed D. Dementia prevalence and care in assisted living. Health Aff (Millwood). 2014;33(4):658–66. https://doi.org/10.1377/hlthaff.2013.1255.
33. Resnick B, Galik E, Boltz M, et al. Polypharmacy in Assisted Living and Impact on Clinical Outcomes. *Consult Pharm*. Jun 1 2018;33(6):321–330. doi:10.4140/TCP.n.2018.321.
34. Hoben M, Hogan DB, Poss JW, et al. Comparing quality of care outcomes between assisted living and nursing homes before and during the COVID-19 pandemic. J Am Geriatr Soc Nov 2023;71(11):3467–3479. doi:https://doi.org/10.1111/jgs.18499.
35. Zhai Y, Yin S, Zhang D. Association between Antipsychotic Drugs and Mortality in Older Persons with Alzheimer's Disease: A Systematic Review and Meta-Analysis. *J Alzheimers Dis*. Mar 31 2016;52(2):631–9. doi:10.3233/jad-151207.
36. Kales HC, Kim HM, Zivin K, et al. Risk of mortality among individual antipsychotics in patients with dementia. Am J Psychiatry Jan 2012;169(1):71–79. doi:https://doi.org/10.1176/appi.ajp.2011.11030347.
37. Ralph SJ, Espinet AJ. Increased All-Cause Mortality by Antipsychotic Drugs: Updated Review and Meta-Analysis in Dementia and General Mental Health Care. *J Alzheimers Dis Rep*. Feb 2 2018;2(1):1–26. doi:10.3233/adr-170042.
38. Kheirbek RE, Fokar A, Little JT, et al. Association between antipsychotics and all-cause mortality among community-dwelling older adults. J Gerontol A Biol Sci Med Sci. 2019;74(12):1916–21. https://doi.org/10.1093/gerona/glz045.
39. Caffrey C, Sengupta M, Park-Lee E, Moss A, Rosenoff E, Harris-Kojetin L. Residents living in residential care facilities: United States, 2010. NCHS Data Brief. 2012;91:1.
40. Kistler CE, Zimmerman S, Ward KT, Reed D, Golin C, Lewis CL. Health of older adults in assisted living and implications for preventive care. Gerontologist. 2017;57(5):949–54. https://doi.org/10.1093/geront/gnw053.
41. Zimmerman S, Guo W, Mao Y, Li Y, Temkin-Greener H. Health care needs in assisted living: survey data may underestimate chronic conditions. J Am Med Dir Assoc. 2021;22(2):471–3. https://doi.org/10.1016/j.jamda.2020.11.036.
42. Freedman VA, Spillman BC. The residential continuum from home to nursing home: size, characteristics and unmet needs of older adults. J Gerontol B Psychol Sci Soc Sci. 2014;69 Suppl 1(Suppl 1):S42–50. https://doi.org/10.1093/geronb/gbu120.
43. Temkin-Greener H, Mao Y, Li Y, McGarry B. Using Medicare Enrollment Data to Identify Beneficiaries in Assisted Living. *J Am Med Dir Assoc*. Feb 20 2022;S1doi:10.1016/j.jamda.2022.01.062.
44. Zan H, Wu Y, Luo Y, Barile JP, Holmes JR, Agner J. Home settings are associated with less functional decline among older adults compared to community-care foster homes and skilled nursing facilities in Hawaii. PLoS One. 2025;20(6):e0326944. https://doi.org/10.1371/journal.pone.0326944.

45. Office of the Assistant Secretary for Planning and Evaluation. Understanding the Characteristics of Older Adults in Different Residential Settings: Data Sources and Trends. Accessed July 2, 2025, https://aspe.hhs.gov/reports/understanding-characteristics-older-adults-different-residential-settings-data-sources-trends-0
46. Bartley MM, Quigg SM, Chandra A, Takahashi PY. Health Outcomes From Assisted Living Facilities: A Cohort Study of a Primary Care Practice. *J Am Med Dir Assoc*. Mar 2018;19(3)doi:10.1016/j.jamda.2017.12.079.
47. Zimmerman S, Sloane PD, Reed D. Dementia prevalence and care in assisted living. Health Aff (Millwood) 2014/04/01 2014;33(4):658–666. doi:https://doi.org/10.1377/hlthaff.2013.1255.
48. Manly JJ, Jones RN, Langa KM, et al. Estimating the prevalence of dementia and mild cognitive impairment in the US: the 2016 health and retirement study harmonized cognitive assessment protocol project. JAMA Neurol. 2022;79(12):1242–9. https://doi.org/10.1001/jamaneurol.2022.3543.
49. Klicnik I, Leadbetter B, Zdjelar M, Bouchard DR, Copeland JL, Dogra S. Inactivity is isolation: insights from a sedentary time intervention in assisted living. *BMC Geriatr*. Apr 25 2025;25(1):281. doi:10.1186/s12877-025-05921-w.
50. Hoben M, Dampf H, Devkota R, et al. Facility-level variation of resident loneliness in assisted living and associated organizational context factors: a repeated cross-sectional study. Int J Geriatr Psychiatry. 2025;40(5):e70093. https://doi.org/10.1002/gps.70093.
51. Lertsuwan K, Soonthornchaiya R, Bunthumporn N. Effects of a meaning in life enhancement program on depression among older adult residents of assisted living facilities. Geriatr Nurs Jan-Feb. 2025;61:287–92. https://doi.org/10.1016/j.gerinurse.2024.11.015.
52. Kolster A, Rautiainen LJ, Aalto UL, et al. The importance of nature and wishes for nature-based experiences among older adults in assisted living facilities. Geriatr Nurs May-Jun. 2025;63:300–6. https://doi.org/10.1016/j.gerinurse.2025.03.061.
53. Holmes SD, Scherr S, O'Brien E, Levy S, Galik E, Resnick B. The meaningful engagement assessment for residents with dementia in assisted living settings. J Am Med Dir Assoc. 2025;26(1):105354. https://doi.org/10.1016/j.jamda.2024.105354.
54. Loomer L, Dauner KN. A Qualitative Analysis of Safety Culture in Minnesota's Assisted Living Facilities. *Gerontologist*. May 10 2025;65(6)doi:10.1093/geront/gnaf119.
55. Wang J, Liebel DV, Yu F, Caprio TV, Shang J. Inverse dose-response relationship between home health care Services and rehospitalization in older adults. J Am Med Dir Assoc. 2018; https://doi.org/10.1016/j.jamda.2018.10.021.
56. Şahin E, Yavuz Veizi BG, Naharci MI. Telemedicine interventions for older adults: a systematic review. J Telemed Telecare. 2024;30(2):305–19. https://doi.org/10.1177/1357633x211058340.
57. Rentscher KE, Klopack ET, Crimmins EM, Seeman TE, Cole SW, Carroll JE. Social relationships and epigenetic aging in older adulthood: results from the health and retirement study. Brain Behav Immun 2023/11/01/ 2023;114:349–359. doi:https://doi.org/https://doi.org/10.1016/j.bbi.2023.09.001.
58. Shippee TP, Akosionu-DeSouza O, Beebe TJ, Parikh RR, Brasure M. Measurement of quality in assisted living in The United States of America: a scoping review. J Am Med Dir Assoc. 2025;26(1):105355. https://doi.org/10.1016/j.jamda.2024.105355.
59. Sloane PD, Zimmerman S, Gruber-Baldini AL, Hebel JR, Magaziner J, Konrad TR. Health and functional outcomes and health care utilization of persons with dementia in residential care and assisted living facilities: comparison with nursing homes. Gerontologist. 2005;45 Spec No 1(1):124-32 https://doi.org/10.1093/geront/45.suppl_1.124.
60. Cornell PY, Zhang W, Thomas KS. Changes in long-term care markets: assisted living supply and the prevalence of low-care residents in nursing homes. J Am Med Dir Assoc. 2020;21(8):1161–1165.e4. https://doi.org/10.1016/j.jamda.2020.01.006.
61. Silver BC, Grabowski DC, Gozalo PL, Dosa D, Thomas KS. Increasing prevalence of assisted living as a substitute for private-pay long-term nursing care. Health Serv Res. 2018;53(6):4906–20. https://doi.org/10.1111/1475-6773.13021.
62. Binette J, Farago F. *Home and community preferences survey: a national survey of adults age 18-plus*. 2024. AARP Research; 2024. Accessed July 3, 2025. https://doi.org/10.26419/res.00831.001

63. Chyr LC, Drabo EF, Fabius CD. Patterns and predictors of transitions across residential care settings and nursing homes among community-dwelling older adults in the United States. Gerontologist. 2020;60(8):1495–503. https://doi.org/10.1093/geront/gnaa070.
64. Manis DR, Kirkwood D, Li W, et al. Clinical and sociodemographic characteristics of new residents of assisted living: a nested case-control study. J Am Med Dir Assoc Nov 2024;25(11):105270. doi:https://doi.org/10.1016/j.jamda.2024.105270.
65. Kabayama M, Mikami H, Kamide K. Factors associated with risk for assisted living among community-dwelling older Japanese. Arch Gerontol Geriatr Jul-Aug. 2016;65:63–9. https://doi.org/10.1016/j.archger.2016.03.005.
66. Becker M, Boaz T, Andel R, DeMuth A. Predictors of avoidable hospitalizations among assisted living residents. J Am Med Dir Assoc. 2012;13(4):355–9. https://doi.org/10.1016/j.jamda.2011.02.001.
67. Grabowski DC, Caudry DJ, Dean KM, Stevenson DG. Integrated payment and delivery models offer opportunities and challenges for residential care facilities. Health Aff (Millwood) 2015/10/01 2015;34(10):1650–1656. doi:https://doi.org/10.1377/hlthaff.2015.0330.
68. Aclan R, George S, Block H, Lane R, Laver K. Middle aged and older adult's perspectives of their own home environment: a review of qualitative studies and meta-synthesis. BMC Geriatr 2023/10/31 2023;23(1):707. doi:https://doi.org/10.1186/s12877-023-04279-1.
69. Roy N, Dubé R, Després C, Freitas A, Légaré F. Choosing between staying at home or moving: a systematic review of factors influencing housing decisions among frail older adults. PLoS One. 2018;13(1):e0189266. https://doi.org/10.1371/journal.pone.0189266.
70. Kemp CL, Ball MM, Morgan JC, Burgess EO, Doyle PJ, Perkins MM. FAMILY INVOLVEMENT IS THE KEY: INFORMAL CARE IN ASSISTED LIVING. *Innovation in* Aging 2017;1(suppl_1):1265-1266. doi:https://doi.org/10.1093/geroni/igx004.4609.
71. Kerpershoek L, Woods B, Wolfs C, et al. Do caregiver profiles predict the use of dementia care services? Findings from the Actifcare study. Aging Ment Health 2018:1–8. doi:https://doi.org/10.1080/13607863.2018.1544215.
72. Villapando MV. Lightening the load: an overview of caregiver burden in dementia care. Home healthcare now. Apr 2015;33(4):190–6.; quiz 197-8. https://doi.org/10.1097/nhh.0000000000000223.
73. Tate K, Hoben M, Grabusic C, Bailey S, Cummings GG. The Association of Service use and Other Client Factors with the time to transition from home care to facility-based care. J Am Med Dir Assoc. 2022;23(1):133–140.e3. https://doi.org/10.1016/j.jamda.2021.06.027.
74. Hua CL, Smith L, Zimmerman S, et al. Admission and discharge practices among assisted living communities: the role of state regulations and organizational characteristics. Gerontologist. 2024;64(8)doi:10.1093/geront/gnae076
75. Mitty E, Flores S. Assisted living nursing practice: admission assessment. Geriatr Nurs. Jan-Feb. 2007;28(1):27–30. https://doi.org/10.1016/j.gerinurse.2006.11.013.
76. Sun C, Ding Y, Cui Y, et al. The adaptation of older adults' transition to residential care facilities and cultural factors: a meta-synthesis. BMC Geriatr 2021/01/18 2021;21(1):64. doi:https://doi.org/10.1186/s12877-020-01987-w.
77. Mueller KE, Van Puymbroeck M, Crowe BM, Davis NJ. Exploring constraints to Well-being for older adults in transition into an assisted living home: a qualitative study. Canadian Journal on Aging / La Revue canadienne du vieillissement. 2023;42(4):688–95. https://doi.org/10.1017/S0714980823000284.
78. Lam K, Harrison JD, Haller L, et al. "nobody can be equipped for this": advice from new residents of long-term care facilities. J Am Geriatr Soc. 2025;73(5):1506–16. https://doi.org/10.1111/jgs.19405.
79. Polacsek M, Woolford M. Strategies to support older adults' mental health during the transition into residential aged care: a qualitative study of multiple stakeholder perspectives. BMC Geriatr 2022/02/24 2022;22(1):151. doi:https://doi.org/10.1186/s12877-022-02859-1.
80. Bradshaw SA, Playford ED, Riazi A. Living well in care homes: a systematic review of qualitative studies. Age Ageing. 2012;41(4):429–40. https://doi.org/10.1093/ageing/afs069.

81. Phillips LJ, Leary E, Blankenship J, Zimmerman S. Physical function, relocation, and mortality outcomes in residential care and assisted living residents. J Aging Health. 2019;31(6):903–24. https://doi.org/10.1177/0898264317740047.
82. Ajay D, Cai S, Guo W, Temkin-Greener H. Urinary incontinence is an independent risk factor for nursing home placement among assisted living residents. J Am Med Dir Assoc. 2025;26(4):105476. https://doi.org/10.1016/j.jamda.2024.105476.
83. Kenny AM, Bellantonio S, Fortinsky RH, et al. Factors associated with skilled nursing facility transfers in dementia-specific assisted living. Alzheimer Dis Assoc Disord Jul-Sep. 2008;22(3):255–60. https://doi.org/10.1097/WAD.0b013e31816c92d5.
84. Dys S, Smith L, Tunalilar O, Carder P. Revisiting the role of physicians in assisted living and residential care settings. Gerontol Geriatr Med Jan-Dec. 2020;6:2333721420979840. https://doi.org/10.1177/2333721420979840.
85. Son JY, Marriott DJ, Struble LM, Chen W, Larson JL. Factors associated with transfer from assisted living facilities to a nursing home: National Health Aging Trends Study 2011-2019. J Am Geriatr Soc Nov 2024;72(11):3374–3384. doi:https://doi.org/10.1111/jgs.19147.
86. Nazareno J, Zhang W, Silver B, Dosa D, Gozalo P, Thomas K. Home health utilization in assisted living settings. Med Care Res Rev. 2019:1077558719835049. https://doi.org/10.1177/1077558719835049.
87. Cornell PY, Gadkari G, Hua CL, et al. Risk of hospitalization among assisted living residents dually enrolled in Medicare and Medicaid. J Am Med Dir Assoc. 2025;26(2):105421. https://doi.org/10.1016/j.jamda.2024.105421.
88. Temkin-Greener H, Mao Y, McGarry B, Zimmerman S, Li Y. Healthcare use and outcomes in assisted living communities: race, ethnicity, and dual eligibility [in press]. Med Care Res Rev. 2021;
89. Hua CL, Nelson I, Cornell PY, White EM, Thomas KS. Changes in nursing staff levels and injury-related emergency department visits among assisted living residents with Alzheimers disease and related dementias. J Am Med Dir Assoc. 2024;25(8):105087. https://doi.org/10.1016/j.jamda.2024.105087.
90. Stearns SC, Park J, Zimmerman S, Gruber-Baldini AL, Konrad TR, Sloane PD. Determinants and effects of nurse staffing intensity and skill mix in residential care/assisted living settings. Gerontologist. 2007;47(5):662–71. https://doi.org/10.1093/geront/47.5.662.
91. Manis DR, Kirkwood D, Fisher S, et al. Transitions to nursing homes among residents of assisted living and community-dwelling home care recipients. J Am Med Dir Assoc. 2025;26(2):105429. https://doi.org/10.1016/j.jamda.2024.105429.
92. Unruh MA, Carney JK, Moreno A, Snyder SL. Optimizing ethical care, quality, and safety in long-term Services and supports: a position paper from the American College of Physicians. Ann Intern Med. 2025;178(6):839–46. https://doi.org/10.7326/annals-24-03641.
93. Bowers LA. Choose: Medical or social model. Mace says December. 2022;5. https://www.mcknightsseniorliving.com/home/news/choose-medical-or-social-model-mace-says/
94. Klinger JH. The changing landscape of assisted living. Updated March 13. December 5, 2022:2018. https://www.pioneernetwork.net/the-changing-landscape-of-assisted-living/
95. Hogan DB, Maxwell CJ, Dampf H, et al. Excess deaths in assisted living and nursing homes during the COVID-19 pandemic in Alberta, Canada. J Am Med Dir Assoc. 2024;25(7):105032. https://doi.org/10.1016/j.jamda.2024.105032.

Chapter 3
State Regulations and Oversight in Assisted Living

Wenhan Guo and Helena Temkin-Greener

Introduction

Assisted living communities represent a unique and a growing sector of long-term residential care [1], designed to provide personal and supportive services to individuals needing assistance due to physical and/or cognitive impairments.[1] These communities began to grow in popularity in the 1980s, in part in response to consumer dissatisfaction with the institutional nature of nursing homes. By comparison, assisted living promised a less restrictive, more home-like environment with greater personal autonomy and a higher quality of life. To fulfill this promise, early assisted living advocates were opposed to strict government regulations [2], arguing they would stifle the flexibility of the model and its focus on residents' autonomy [3]. Over time, while nursing homes became increasingly more regulated, operating under stringent federal and state guidelines, state regulation of assisted living also grew, but due to variation across the country has been described by some as a "state-level patchwork," [4] reflecting approaches ranging from comprehensive licensing and regulatory frameworks to those that are less specific. Nonetheless, progress has been made over the last 25 years, when there was national concern about lax regulation and oversight [5].

As assisted living communities gained in popularity, concerns about the lack of specific standards of care and resident safety became more common. As a result of the

[1] Assisted living communities serve older adults who are no longer able to live independently in the community, although some also serve younger people with intellectual disabilities or mental illness. The focus of this chapter is on the communities that serve older adults.

W. Guo (✉)
Ohio University, Athens, OH, USA
e-mail: wenhan@ohio.edu

H. Temkin-Greener
University of Rochester, Rochester, NY, USA
e-mail: Helena_Temkin-Greener@urmc.rochester.edu

H. Temkin-Greener and S. Zimmerman (eds.), *Assisted Living Through Research, Policy, and Practice*, https://doi.org/10.1007/978-3-032-32088-9_3

April 2001 hearing held by the U.S. Senate Special Committee on Aging, the National Assisted Living Workgroup was convened to establish guidelines and recommendations for assisted living policies nationwide [6]. The workgroup endorsed over 100 recommendations for best practices, with the consensus of the meeting being that the industry would work to self-regulate, with states maintaining regulatory authority [6]. By 2019, over 2250 regulations consistent with the workgroup's recommendations were in effect [3], but states differed widely in whether and how they regulated direct care in assisted living [4]. At the same time, few states promulgated regulations impacting residents' rights, staffing levels and training, or medication management [4]. As the needs of assisted living residents have become more complex, some state regulations have not always kept pace, while others regularly update their regulations. From July 1, 2023 to July 1, 2024, fifteen states reported regulatory/legislative updates [7]. For example, 25 states now have some quality measurement data collection or management requirements and 45 states have implemented new infection control requirements for assisted living communities [7].

Similar to all regulations, state assisted living regulations are meant to set the floor for the care practices and operations of these communities. The extent to which assisted living communities exceed state regulations is not clear due to lack of data. However, recent research has shown that the quality of care provided in assisted living communities, as measured by place of death and end-of-life care transitions, is strongly associated with the specificity[2] of the base regulations established at the state level [8, 9]. In this chapter we examine variations in assisted living regulations, compliance, and enforcement, and their associations with consumers' care access and quality.

To Regulate or Not and How Much?

The origins of regulation in long-term care can be traced back to the mid-twentieth century when the federal government established oversight mechanisms for nursing homes under Medicare and Medicaid [10]. In the 1960s and 1970s, numerous investigations revealed widespread quality of care issues in nursing homes across the US including systematic over-medication, inadequate staffing, and instances of resident abuse [11]. These issues led to public outrage and demands for increased oversight of long-term care facilities [11]. Public awareness and advocacy for stronger regulations culminated with a comprehensive report on nursing home quality released by the Institute of Medicine in 1986 [12], which was followed by the 1987 Nursing Home Reform Act, mandating stricter regulations and higher standards of care [13, 14]. These efforts focused on nursing homes and they likely had little or no significant

[2] Specificity (sometimes referred to as stringency) of regulations is a concept used by researchers to indicate the level of detail in the regulations. For example, some states do not specify the minimum number of direct care workers required to be on site while others require staff to be present in proportion to the number of the residents; with the latter conveying higher regulatory specificity (or greater stringency).

impact on assisted living given that these communities were still somewhat nascent at the time.

While many nursing home experts consider regulation essential, they are aware of their limitations, including often excessive administrative burden for the nursing home or loss of autonomy/flexibility for the residents that may result in fixed schedules and lack of person-centered care [15, 16]. In assisted living, controversy around regulations may be even more pronounced and complex. Because these communities represent a variety of care models, range in size, and operate under different license classifications [17], determining the right regulatory fit to assure safety yet permit person-centered care—thus achieving a balance between "assisted" and "living" [18] — is akin to Goldilocks' dilemma of finding the middle ground. This dilemma may involve several key tensions such as *safety* vs *autonomy* or *standardization* vs *person-centered care*. For example, regulations that involve strict safety measures vis-à-vis medication management may aim to protect residents' *safety* but effectively may limit their *autonomy* to control their medications. Similarly, regulations requiring certain care *standards* may assure similar care practices across communities, but may prevent the residents from experiencing a "home-like" environment that focuses on *person-centered care*. Finding the balance between the necessary structure and safety guidelines while allowing flexibility to promote residents' well-being and independence is the proverbial Goldilocks' dilemma.

The premise of assisted living lies in its focus on personal supportive services (*assistance*) being provided to maximize residents' person-centered care (independence, privacy, and choice) and minimize the need to move elsewhere (*living*). When residents' safety and clinical oversight are prioritized, stricter regulations may be favored. For example, consumers may advocate for stricter regulations as important for better quality of care and the protection of residents' rights [3]. Insurers and financial underwriters may favor more specific state regulations (such as related to staffing) [3, 19]. States with a higher proportion of Medicaid-eligible older beneficiaries residing in assisted living communities may also require more stringent regulations, at least in some domains (e.g., admission and retention) [20]. At the same time, assisted living owners/operators may have incentives to favor more permissive regulatory environments, particularly regarding staffing and service delivery standards, as stricter regulations can intensify competition for a limited workforce and impose compliance costs that challenge operational viability [21, 22]. Those favoring fewer regulations caution that stricter policies may undermine access to assisted living or prevent aging in place, for example when they do not allow admission/re-entry or mandate discharge for residents with certain conditions (e.g., with pressure ulcers or in need of skilled nursing care) [18, 23]. In place of stricter regulations, some may favor negotiated risk agreements, in which residents and/or families acknowledge and agree to accept the risks associated with certain preferred behaviors or activities (e.g., walking without being accompanied), and a priori accept any resulting and potentially negative consequences.

Federal Oversight

Assisted living communities continue to grow in popularity, with recent reports citing over one million residents; 80% of whom are 75 years of age or older [24]. Unlike nursing homes, which must ensure compliance with federal regulations of residents' rights, quality assurance, performance improvement, quality measures and their reporting, assisted living remains largely exempt from federal oversight because Medicare does not cover assisted living services. However, Medicaid, while not covering room and board, does pay for some medical and non-medical services provided in assisted living, allowing for some federal oversight of these communities. Medicaid services are covered largely through Home and Community-Based Services (HCBS) programs, and because the federal government approves these waivers, states must follow federal requirements for their administration [23]. Assisted living operators must also follow other federal policies, not specific to assisted living, such as those promulgated by the Fair Housing Act, the Americans with Disabilities Act, and others [3]. Overall, federal oversight of assisted living communities is indirect and relies mainly on state actions and reporting requirements [25].

State Oversight

State regulations governing assisted living fall into several broad categories that cover licensing and certification, staffing and training, scope of services, health and safety standards, resident rights, financial transparency and billing, and enforcement. In each of these categories, regulations vary across states, and sometimes within states, with respect to what is regulated and the specificity of the regulations. These variations reflect differences in how states conceptualize assisted living, the populations they seek to protect, and the balance they attempt to strike between safety, autonomy, and flexibility. In the sections below, we describe these key regulatory domains and examine how variations in regulations may be associated with differences in service use and residents' outcomes.

Licensing and Certification

Assisted living regulation (licensing) and certification processes are related, yet are quite different. Licensure is a mandatory, legal authorization granted by a state that allows an assisted living community to operate. Non-compliance may lead to fines, inability to admit residents, suspension or revocation of license, or closure. In most states, assisted living communities are required to renew their licenses annually or bi-annually, but some states permit longer renewal periods of up to three years [21,

26]. License renewals may or may not involve inspections to ensure compliance with standards [17].

Certification is typically a voluntary designation or recognition that a provider meets specialized standards for services beyond baseline licensure. Certification may be optional unless it is required to provide a specific service, for example, to operate a memory care unit. Some states use the word certification for what is effectively a regulatory process (e.g., "certified assisted living"). Thus the key difference between regulation and certification is whether it is required to legally operate and whether it is enforced under state law.

All states require assisted living communities to be licensed, but the criteria and processes vary widely. In some states, such as California and Florida, licensing is highly structured with guidelines regarding care standards, staffing requirements, and building safety [21, 27, 28]. Other states may focus broadly on health and safety standards without providing much detail. [21, 29]. Some states differentiate assisted living into multiple categories or certification levels (e.g., New York) [30, 31], while others (e.g., California) license a single primary type [29, 32]. Many states require a separate license or designation for memory care units [29]. Furthermore, special levels of certification based on a higher standard of care may be required in some states (e.g., Ohio), particularly when Medicaid or Medicare reimbursable services such as personal care or physical therapy are provided by a certified agency to a qualified resident [33, 34].

A recent study identified 182 license classifications for assisted living across the US, with multiple primary types, subtypes, and designations [29]. While this study confirmed variations in licensing and certification between states, it also pointed out significant within-state variations [29]. State sublicenses designed to protect subgroups of residents, for example those in dementia-memory care settings, may require staff in these units to have dementia-specific training, yet such training may not be required of staff serving residents with dementia who are not living in memory-care units. Given the assisted living population growth among residents with dementia who do not reside in memory care [35], these may be significant omissions in the states' regulatory processes. Furthermore, dementia-care regulations are also highly variable. One study identified several dementia-care policies (e.g., preadmission assessment, consumer disclosure, dementia-staffing and training, building design) and found that on average fewer than half of these policies were included in state regulations, ranging from none in Hawaii to almost all in Arkansas and Illinois [20].

In states with rigorous regulatory processes, assisted living communities are typically required to demonstrate compliance with a range of standards before opening [17]. These processes include building codes, fire safety measures, sanitary requirements, and health and safety inspections. Regulations also often involve detailed requirements for staff qualifications, including education and training prior to the employment start date, and for continuing education [17].

Staffing and Training

Both staffing and staff training focus on areas of practice that directly impact quality of care provided to the residents [20, 36]. Regulations also specify the level of care that communities may provide which have implications for staffing, including restrictions on the provision of skilled nursing care or medication administration [20, 36, 37]. A recent study examined stringency of state assisted living regulations in various domains, one being staffing and training [20]. For each state, and each regulatory domain, stringency scores were calculated with higher scores indicating greater stringency. For the four staffing/training regulations that were assessed—direct care worker (DCW) day and overnight staffing, licensed staffing, DCW training, in-service training—the average stringency score across all states was 61%, ranging from 32% in New Hampshire to 87% in Pennsylvania and Virginia [20].

On-site licensed nursing and access to medical care are also unevenly regulated across states. While some states mandate the availability of licensed nurses during certain hours or require communities to contract with on-call physicians, others permit communities to operate with unlicensed staff and minimal or no clinical oversight. A study that examined the relationship between the specificity of assisted living staffing regulations and resident hospitalizations found that in states which increased the specificity of their direct care worker staffing from "sufficient" to "ratio proportional to residents," there was an overall 4% reduction in hospital risk and a 6% reduction of risk among residents with dementia; conversely, a similar change in regulatory specificity for licensed nurses was associated with a 2.5% and a 5% increase in hospitalizations overall and among residents with dementia, respectively [36]. This evidence points to possibly unintended consequences of increased specificity in staffing regulations. Increasing direct care worker staffing specificity may mean fewer adverse events (e.g., falls) among the residents, thus fewer hospitalizations, whereas increasing licensed nurse staffing may mean there is greater ability to detect clinical changes among residents that may prompt their hospitalizations. Alternatively, these findings may indicate staff substitution in which requirements for higher staffing or more expensive personnel (licensed nurses) is offset by reducing the less expensive labor, thus leading to more hospitalizations. Whichever explanation is the "right one," changes in staffing regulations and their specificity may have downstream consequences to assisted living communities and their residents.

Other studies showed statistically significant positive associations between greater regulatory staffing and training specificity and better end-of-life quality of care outcomes, including fewer care transitions and higher probability of dying in the assisted living community (i.e., at home) [8, 9]. Together, these studies point out the complexities in state assisted living regulations and the associated (but not necessarily causal) relationships that are not always intended as regulatory specificity is lowered or increased.

Although all states mandate some level of training for assisted living staff, the specifics, including the number of training hours, educational content, and qualifications of the trainers, differ widely [20, 21]. Some states have comprehensive training programs that emphasize dementia care, infection control, and emergency response, while others impose only minimal requirements [21, 38, 39]. For instance, Massachusetts requires assisted living staff to complete 54 hours of initial training before working with residents [40]. This training encompasses topics such as personal care, aging, nutrition, medication management, and emergency procedures [40]. Additionally, staff must undergo ongoing annual training, including 10 hours of education with at least 2 hours focused on dementia care. Employees in special care residences are required to complete an additional 4 hours of training annually related to residents' specialized care needs [40]. Although staff training is generally more regulated than other aspects of assisted living care [20, 36], questions remain about whether current requirements are sufficient to meet the increasingly complex care needs of the residents, particularly as more individuals with chronic conditions and cognitive impairments take up residence in assisted living [3, 41]. For example, one recent study reported that staff often lack sufficient training in critical areas such as dementia care or care for people with complex needs [18].

Scope of Services

Assisted living communities are generally required by state regulations to provide the following services: room and board, with housekeeping; typically 3 meals daily; assistance with activities of daily living (e.g., bathing, dressing, grooming); availability of staff 24/7; emergency call system; transportation; and social and recreational activities and supports [42]. Assisted living providers may also directly offer or arrange for personal care services and specialized care such as provided in memory care units.

Services that assisted living communities are allowed to provide to their residents are closely regulated [20]. Some states permit assisted living communities to offer comprehensive medical and skilled nursing services, while others restrict services to personal care and assistance with daily activities [20, 41]. For instance, Minnesota allows assisted living communities to provide a broad range of services, including nursing care and medication management, under its licensure framework established in 2021 [26]. New York restricts services in assisted living to non-medical assistance, requiring that residents needing skilled nursing care transition to licensed nursing facilities [43].

Regulations concerning medication management are notably inconsistent across states. While some states allow trained unlicensed staff to administer medications, others require licensed nursing professionals for such tasks [20, 21, 44]. In Florida, trained but unlicensed assistant-level personnel may help residents with self-administration of medications, provided they complete specific training programs[45]. On the other hand, Massachusetts mandates that only licensed nurses administer medications, reflecting a more medicalized and regulated model of service delivery [46]. These differences may directly impact resident safety and medication adherence, potentially increasing the risk of medication errors and adverse health events if medications are not taken as directed due to lack of assistance [47, 48].

Health and Safety Standards

Health and safety regulations are intended to ensure the well-being of assisted living residents, many of whom are frail, have multiple chronic conditions, and may be living with cognitive impairment [9, 35, 49]. While certain domains such as fire safety, emergency preparedness, and sanitation are more clearly regulated [18], others, like infection control, remain less regulated and less enforced [38, 39].

The Centers for Medicare & Medicaid Services (CMS) Life Safety Code outlines national fire safety requirements for health care facilities, including assisted living communities, that receive federal funding or are co-located with Medicare-certified entities [50]. These requirements include standards and regulations for smoke alarms, sprinkler systems, fire drills, and egress planning [50]. In most states, adherence to these codes is mandatory and subject to periodic inspections [50]. Similarly, requirements for sanitation, including those for kitchen cleanliness, water quality, and waste disposal, are often explicitly regulated, echoing long-standing public health concerns that preceded the existence of modern assisted living models [51–53].

Emergency preparedness—including evacuation planning, back up of power supply, and staff training for disaster response—is an area in which assisted living regulations are generally quite comprehensive [54]. In the wake of natural disasters and public health emergencies such as Hurricane Katrina and the COVID-19 pandemic, there has been more attention paid to this regulatory domain in long-term care settings [3, 55, 56]. However, unlike nursing homes, many assisted living communities are not subject to federal emergency preparedness requirements unless they are co-located with Medicare-certified providers [57]. A 2022 survey of state agencies responsible for assisted living oversight indicated that in half of the states, oversight was dispersed across three or more agencies, which at times may contribute to inconsistencies in monitoring and enforcement of emergency preparedness standards [58]. The COVID-19 pandemic exposed some such vulnerabilities, with assisted living communities reporting lack of resources (e.g., personal protective equipment - PPE), staffing shortages, and inadequate staff training to effectively contain outbreaks [59, 60]. To date, only a few states have specific regulatory policies addressing PPE, testing, cohorting, or communication during infectious disease outbreaks in assisted living [3].

Enforcement of assisted living state regulations in terms of inspection practices and public reporting also remains variable [17]. A national survey of state monitoring and enforcement agents revealed that while nearly all states conduct inspections at the time of licensure and in response to complaints, fewer conduct routine annual inspections. Only five states engaged in all forms of inspection (licensure, complaint-based, routine, and at-will[3]). Regulations regarding public disclosure of information, including inspections, also vary across states. While two-thirds of states require that notices of violations be posted in a public space in the assisted living community, about one-third require communities to share information of violations with state officials or within the industry. Only 7 states require assisted living communities to submit an annual compliance report. Although budgets to support state assisted living monitoring and licensing have been sparse, a quarter of state agents reported increase in budgets compared to five years prior [58].

In conclusion, health and safety regulations in assisted living reflect a mix of more established and less developed regulatory approaches. Fire safety, sanitation, and structural building standards are generally well regulated and enforced, whereas regulatory domains involving clinical processes, infection prevention, and staff preparedness are less developed and inconsistently regulated across states.

Resident Rights

In long-term residential settings, resident rights are foundational to protecting the dignity, autonomy, and well-being of individuals residing in congregate environments. However, while federal law explicitly outlines a bill of rights for nursing home residents under the 1987 Nursing Home Reform Act 61, there is no corresponding federal framework governing resident rights in assisted living. As a result, regulatory protections for assisted living residents are generally less consistent, often weaker, and shaped primarily at the state level [4]. This "patchwork approach," [4] as some have called it, leads to variations in both the content of residents' rights and the mechanisms available for their enforcement. For example, California mandates explicit rights such as freedom from retaliation due to complaints or the ability to access personal records, whereas other states (e.g., South Carolina) provide only general assurances of "dignity" without specifying enforceable provisions [62].

Because assisted living is licensed at the state level, states develop their own statutes or administrative rules for resident protections. These statutes and rules may be included in assisted living licensing rules or addressed separately through long-term care ombudsman programs [63, 64]. Yet, as noted in the literature, many of the foundational concepts associated with resident rights in assisted living are adopted by reference to rights defined for nursing home residents, such as the right to dignity, privacy, autonomy, and protection from abuse and neglect, rather than developed specifically for the assisted living model [15, 65]. Nevertheless, several rights are broadly recognized across states, as evidenced in official publications by

[3] Complaint-based visits are inspections initiated in response to specific complaints or allegations regarding a community. Routine visits are regularly scheduled inspections that occur at predetermined intervals to assess ongoing compliance. At-will visits are unscheduled inspections initiated at the discretion of the monitoring agency, not necessarily tied to a complaint or routine schedule.

ombudsman programs in states such as Indiana, California, Massachusetts, Ohio, and Texas [63, 64, 66, 67]. These include the right to be treated with dignity and respect, the right to participate in one's own care decisions, the right to privacy and confidentiality, the right to voice grievances without fear of retaliation, the right to manage personal finances, and the right to freedom from abuse and neglect [63, 64, 66, 67]. Additionally, residents generally have the right to have visitors, participate in social and religious activities, and receive written information about community policies and fees, as well as reasons and procedures for discharge [66–68].

Enforcement of these rights remains variable. Unlike nursing homes, assisted living communities do not undergo federally mandated surveys that include resident rights assessments. Instead, oversight is conducted by state surveyors or ombudsman programs, which often are under-resourced and may be limited in their authority. Ombudsmen serve as resident advocates, investigate complaints, mediate disputes, and educate staff and residents about rights and responsibilities [69]. The effectiveness of ombudsman programs varies depending on state funding, staffing, and legal authority [69]. In some states, ombudsmen can enter assisted living communities without notice and have direct access to residents; in others, their access or scope is more limited [63, 68, 69].

Translating residents' rights regulations into day-to-day practice may be challenging. Research shows that residents often perceive their rights to autonomy and self-determination as being constrained by established routines, staffing limitations, or paternalistic attitudes among caregivers [70–72]. While technically residents may be allowed to make choices about meals or bathing times, staff shortages may limit the meaningful exercise of those rights; similarly, the right to refuse care can be complicated by providers' safety concerns, fears of liability, or unclear communication between residents, their family members and staff [71].

In summary, while the concept of resident rights in assisted living is foundational, its practical application may be limited by absence of standards and inconsistent state-level regulations. The ombudsman program remains an important avenue for assuring and advocating for residents' rights, but its effectiveness may be limited by the authority vested in the program and its resources.

Financial Transparency and Billing

Despite the growing reliance on assisted living as a long-term residential option, empirical evidence on financial transparency and billing regulations in this setting remains limited. Most research around financial disclosure, accountability, and affordability in long-term care focuses on the nursing home industry, where federal reimbursement through Medicaid and Medicare triggers more stringent reporting requirements [73–75]. In contrast, the largely private-pay assisted living model creates a regulatory blind spot — one in which consumers navigate different fee structures, pricing models, and billing practices sometimes in absence of a standardized regulatory framework for financial clarity [76].

Prospective residents and their families may encounter a lack of or unclear disclosures about total service cost, fee escalations, and service bundling that may make it difficult to compare assisted living communities or to understand what is and is not included in a base rate [77]. For instance, some communities, such as The Arbors and The Ivy in Massachusetts and Connecticut, respectively, offer all-inclusive pricing that encompasses housing, meals, and personal care services within a single monthly fee [78]. Other communities like Benton House in Florida adopt an à la carte model, where residents pay a base rate for housing and meals, with additional charges for personal care services such as assistance with bathing or medication management, often being billed in 15-minute increments [78, 79]. While many assisted living communities provide clear financial information to their residents, not all states require providers to clearly differentiate between care-related and non-care-related charges [77]. For example, communities may charge separately for assistance with bathing or medication management in addition to housing and meals or they may include all services in one bundled fee, but many states do not require assisted living providers to disclose this information at admission [80, 81]. Some observers suggested that this lack of standardization contributes to both consumer confusion and the potential for billing disputes, although research in this area is sparse and thus inconclusive [76].

Because of potential concerns and the need for financial accountability in long-term residential settings receiving federal reimbursement, nursing homes are required by state and federal legislation to report their ownership structures, financial details regarding companies with which they are affiliated, and the detailed use of public funds [82]. However, the assisted living industry, which shares many of the same risks as does the nursing home sector—limited consumer choice, inequities in access, and diminished trust—has no similar regulatory requirements [3, 41].

Enforcement of Regulations

State regulation of assisted living is important to ensure resident safety and care quality. Unfortunately, research on state regulatory enforcement of assisted living is rather sparse and does not provide a complete or clear picture of the existing enforcement mechanisms and their application. One study on this topic reviewed assisted living financial enforcement penalty structures in 25 states and found substantial differences in how penalties are applied: some states allowed either per-day or per-instance fines, while others limited enforcement to one method; one state had no enforcement regulations at all. The median maximum per-instance fine was $2000, with a median per-day fine of $500. Severity of the fines often depended on past violations or the assessed scope and the severity of the infraction. In only 3 of the 25 surveyed states, enforcement severity was dependent on community size, whereas most states applied the same penalty structure regardless of the size [83]. It is important to note that at least half of assisted living communities are considered small, i.e., having fewer than 25 beds. These smaller communities are also more likely to have higher proportions of residents who are dually entitled to Medicare and Medicaid, often used as a proxy for resource-poorer communities. When state fines are not adjusted for the size of the community they may disproportionately penalize smaller communities while making fines for larger and more affluent communities far less consequential.

The degree to which enforcement leads to improved care outcomes remains largely unexamined as there is little empirical evidence linking enforcement practices to resident outcomes in assisted living. A review of the literature identified this as a significant gap in both policy and academic inquiry [22]. Similarly, the adequacy of current penalties, or whether enforcement actions have a sustained impact on compliance, has remained largely unexamined. Given the growing demand for assisted living and the services they provide to frail older adults, particularly those with dementia or complex care needs, there is a clear need for more research that evaluates enforcement mechanisms and their impact on care practices and outcomes across states.

Implication for "Assisted" and "Living"

For individuals residing in assisted living communities, access to services, health and safety, the protection of rights, and other aspects of communal living may depend not only on the community of residence, but also on the state in which the community is located [20, 83, 84]. While many states have implemented comprehensive regulatory standards for assisted living operations, others have promulgated only minimal standards often lacking in specificity. These regulatory gaps may be particularly problematic as the resident population becomes increasingly complex, with higher rates of cognitive impairment, complex chronic conditions, and the need for end-of-life care. Further, findings from research on the relationship between state assisted living regulations and residents' quality of care and outcomes have been equivocal. Some have shown that in states with more specific direct care worker staffing and training regulations, residents have better outcomes measured by fewer disruptive end-of-life care transitions and longer home-time, i.e., time alive and outside of formal healthcare [9, 85]. Other studies, however, have shown that higher regulatory specificity of licensed nursing staff was associated with more hospitalizations [36], which may or may not be a good outcome. Either way, these studies point out that state regulations likely play a role in how much "assistance" is rendered to assisted living residents [18]. When "assistance" is timely, person-centered, and scope-appropriate, it enables assisted living residents to age in place promoting quality of life ("living"). But as research has shown, stricter state regulations may also have unintended consequences, raising concerns among the proponents as well as the opponents of stricter state regulations.

To assure a better balance between the "assisted" and the "living," providers, state regulators, and consumer advocates may seek to collaboratively develop a national inventory of core regulatory standards to ensure more equitable and consistent care across assisted living communities. Such an inventory might include both minimal and optimal requirements for staff training, clearer guidelines for medication administration, and protections of residents' rights tailored to the assisted living context. Importantly, this suggestion does not mean adopting a rigid, one-size-fits-all model. Instead, this may be a foundation upon which states can build and innovate.

Drawing from the practice of federal oversight of nursing homes—without replicating its more rigid elements—the federal government, working collaboratively with state agencies, could encourage the establishment of national uniform data reporting [86]. Information contained in such a database would allow consumers to make informed decisions when seeking entrance to assisted living, and may also incentivize providers to compete on quality, promoting both "assistance" and "living." Online reviews provided by consumers on platforms such as Google, demonstrate a significant interest in such information among consumers and their family members [78]. Better assisted living online reviews have been shown to be positively associated with better patient-centered measure of home time, as well as with more specific state regulations [85], suggesting that such reviews may already be an important source signaling care quality in these communities.

In addition, states and assisted living providers could work together to allow for a broader use of negotiated risk or service agreements with residents and families to permit residents to enjoy preferred activities while recognizing and accepting the risks that these may entail to themselves and their service providers. Such agreements may be hard to implement, however, particularly when involving individuals with cognitive impairment who may not fully grasp the risks involved in their decisions [87].

The importance of state regulations for staffing and training, and their relationship to care quality, has been demonstrated by several research studies, as have workforce shortages. Permitting assisted living providers to supplement their services with third-party services may create opportunities for more "assistance" and more "living" [18, 88]. Assisted living operators should be able to provide services that consumers need and desire in order to fulfill the promise of "assisted" and "living." At the same time, consumers need sufficient quality information they can trust as to what assistance these communities provide and what quality of living they may expect. Consumers must be informed so as to be able to "vote with their feet" and thus to advocate for better "assistance" and more "living" in assisted living.

Competing Interests
The authors have no conflicts of interest to declare that are relevant to the content of this chapter

References

1. Residential Care Community Resident Characteristics: United States, 2022. https://www.cdc.gov/nchs/data/databriefs/db506.pdf. Accessed May 11, 2025.
2. Brown WK. Historical evolution of assisted living in the United States, 1979 to the present. The Gerontologist. 2007;47(S1):8–22. https://doi.org/10.1093/geront/47.Supplement_1.8.

3. Zimmerman S, Carder P, Schwartz L, et al. The imperative to reimagine assisted living. J Am Med Dir Assoc. 2022;23(2):225–34. https://doi.org/10.1016/j.jamda.2021.12.004.
4. Smith L, Xu L. Patchwork protections: regulatory oversight in assisted Living. Public Policy Aging Rep. 2021;31(2):62–6. https://doi.org/10.1093/ppar/prab006.
5. Assisted Living: Quality-of-Care and Consumer Protection Issues in Four States. Accessed March 26, 2024. https://www.gao.gov/products/hehs-99-27
6. A Report To The U.S. Senate Special Committee On Aging From The assisted living Workgroup. https://theceal.org/wp-content/uploads/2023/01/AssistedLivingWorkgroupReport-April2003-with-appendices.pdf. Accessed May 9, 2025.
7. 2024 NCAL Assisted Living State Regulatory Review. https://www.ahcancal.org/Assisted-Living/Policy/Documents/2024_RegReview_Overview%20and%20Executive%20Summary.pdf Accessed April 3, 2025
8. Temkin-Greener H, Guo W, Hua Y, et al. End-of-life care in assisted living communities: race and ethnicity, dual enrollment status, and state regulations. Health Aff Proj Hope. 2022, 41(5), pp. 654–62. https://doi.org/10.1377/hlthaff.2021.01677
9. Guo W, Cai S, Caprio T, Schwartz L, Temkin-Greener H. End-of-life care transitions in assisted living: associations with state staffing and training regulations. J Am Med Dir Assoc. 2023;24(6):827–832.e3. https://doi.org/10.1016/j.jamda.2023.02.002.
10. Morford TG. Nursing home regulation: history and expectations. Health Care Financ Rev. 1988;1988(Suppl):129–32.
11. Hynes CJ. The regulation of nursing homes: a case study. Proc Acad Polit Sci. 1980;33(4):126–36. https://doi.org/10.2307/1173861.
12. Improving the quality of long-term care. National Academies Press (US); 2001. Accessed January 18, 2025. https://www.ncbi.nlm.nih.gov/books/NBK224501/
13. Hawes C. Elder abuse in residential long-term care settings: what is known and what information is needed? *Elder mistreatment: abuse, neglect, and exploitation in an aging America.* National Academies Press (US); 2003. Accessed January 18, 2025. https://www.ncbi.nlm.nih.gov/books/NBK98786/
14. Werner RM, Konetzka RT, Grabowski DC, Stevenson DG. Reforming nursing home financing, payment, and oversight. N Engl J Med. 2022;386(20):1869–71. https://doi.org/10.1056/NEJMp2203429.
15. The National Imperative to improve nursing home quality: honoring our commitment to residents, families, and staff. National Academies Press (US); 2022. Accessed March 30, 2025. https://www.ncbi.nlm.nih.gov/books/NBK584660/
16. Improving the quality of care in nursing homes. National Academies Press (US); 1986. Accessed March 30, 2025. https://www.ncbi.nlm.nih.gov/books/NBK217553/
17. A guide to assisted living regulations. Accessed January 14, 2025. https://www.aplaceformom.com/caregiver-resources/articles/assisted-living-violations
18. Zimmerman S, Stone R, Carder P, Thomas K. Does assisted living provide assistance and promote living? Health Aff Proj Hope. 2024, 43(5), pp. 674–81. https://doi.org/10.1377/hlthaff.2023.00972
19. Zimmerman S, Sloane PD, Katz PR, Kunze M, O'Neil K, Resnick B. The need to include assisted living in responding to the COVID-19 pandemic. J Am Med Dir Assoc. 2020;21(5):572–5. https://doi.org/10.1016/j.jamda.2020.03.024.
20. Temkin-Greener H, Mao Y, Ladwig S, Cai X, Zimmerman S, Li Y. Variability and potential determinants of assisted living state regulatory stringency. J Am Med Dir Assoc. 2021;22(8):1714–1719.e2. https://doi.org/10.1016/j.jamda.2020.10.014.
21. NCAL Assisted Living State Regulatory Review. Accessed February 15, 2025. https://www.ahcancal.org/Assisted-Living/Policy/Documents/2023_reg_review.pdf
22. Stevenson DG, Grabowski DC. Sizing up the market for assisted living. Health Aff Proj Hope. 2010;29(1):35–43. https://doi.org/10.1377/hlthaff.2009.0527.
23. Pitz L. The Critical Need for State Regulation of Assisted Living Facilities: Defining "Critical Incidents", Implementing Staff Training, and Requiring Disclosure of Facility Data Note. Minn Law Rev 2020;105(2):1009–1052.

24. Assisted Living Facts & Figures. Accessed December 29, 2025. https://www.ahcancal.org/Assisted-Living/Facts-and-Figures/Pages/default.aspx
25. Medicaid Assisted Living Services: Improved Federal Oversight of Beneficiary Health and Welfare is Needed. Accessed March 30, 2025. https://www.gao.gov/products/gao-18-179
26. Assisted Living Licensure - MN Dept. of Health. Accessed May 7, 2025. https://www.health.state.mn.us/facilities/regulation/assistedliving/index.html
27. Chapter 400 Section 23–2003 Florida Statutes - The Florida Senate. Accessed December 29, 2025. https://flsenate.gov/laws/statutes/2003/400.23
28. Residential Care Facilities for the Elderly. Accessed February 7, 2025. https://www.cdss.ca.gov/getinfo/pdf/rcfe1.PDF.
29. Smith L, Carder P, Bucy T, et al. Connecting policy to licensed assisted living communities, introducing health services regulatory analysis. Health Serv Res. 2021;56(3):540–9. https://doi.org/10.1111/1475-6773.13616.
30. New York Codes, Rules and Regulations. Title 10, Part 1001, §1001.5. Applications for Licensure as an Assisted Living Residence; Certification as Enhanced Assisted Living and Special Needs Assisted Living. Accessed December 9, 2025. https://regulations.justia.com/states/new-york/title-10/chapter-x/part-1001/section-1001-5/
31. New York Codes, Rules and regulations. Title 10, §1001.2. Accessed December 9, 2025. https://www.law.cornell.edu/regulations/new-york/10-NYCRR-1001.2
32. California Code of Regulations. Title 22, Divisions 2 and 6. Online California Code of Regulations. Accessed December 29, 2025. https://www.cdss.ca.gov/inforesources/letters-regulations/legislation-and-regulations/community-care-licensing-regulations/residential
33. Fabius CD, Cornell PY, Zhang W, Thomas KS. State Medicaid financing and access to large assisted living settings for Medicare-Medicaid dual-eligibles. Med Care Res Rev MCRR. 2022;79(1):69–77. https://doi.org/10.1177/1077558720987666.
34. Ohio Administrative Code. Rule 173–39-02.16. Accessed December 23, 2025. https://codes.ohio.gov/ohio-administrative-code/rule-173-39-02.16
35. ALC Facts & Figures. Accessed February 14, 2022. https://www.ahcancal.org/Assisted-Living/Facts-and-Figures/Pages/default.aspx
36. Thomas KS, Cornell PY, Zhang W, et al. The relationship between states' staffing regulations and hospitalizations of assisted living residents. Health Aff (Millwood). 2021;40(9):1377–85. https://doi.org/10.1377/hlthaff.2021.00598.
37. State Regulatory Provisions for Residential Care Settings: An Overview of Staffing Requirements. Accessed March 8, 2025. https://www.rti.org/sites/default/files/resources/State_Regulatory_Provisions_for_Residential_Care_Settings.pdf.
38. Kossover RA, Chi CJ, Wise ME, Tran AH, Chande ND, Perz JF. Infection prevention and control standards in assisted living facilities: are residents' needs being met? J Am Med Dir Assoc. 2014;15(1):47–53. https://doi.org/10.1016/j.jamda.2013.09.011.
39. Mitty E. Infection control practices in assisted living communities. Geriatr Nur (Lond). 2009;30(6):417–23. https://doi.org/10.1016/j.gerinurse.2009.09.008.
40. Training Requirements of Assisted Living Residence Staff. Accessed May 7, 2025. https://www.mass.gov/info-details/training-requirements-of-assisted-living-residence-staff
41. Katz PR, Howd S, Rust C. Reimagining medical care in assisted living. J Am Med Dir Assoc. 2022;23(2):201–3. https://doi.org/10.1016/j.jamda.2021.12.012.
42. State Regulatory Resources. Accessed December 29, 2025. https://www.ahcancal.org/Assisted-Living/Policy/Pages/state-regulations.aspx
43. New York State Department of Health. Adult Care Facilities/assisted living. Accessed May 7, 2025. https://www.health.ny.gov/facilities/adult_care/
44. Mitty E. Medication management in assisted living: a national survey of policies and practices. J Am Med Dir Assoc. 2009;10(2):107–14. https://doi.org/10.1016/j.jamda.2008.08.006.
45. Chapter 429 Section 256–2024 Florida Statutes. Accessed May 7, 2025. https://www.flsenate.gov/laws/statutes/2024/429.256
46. Massachusetts Code of Regulations. 651 CMR §12.04. General Requirements for an assisted living Residence. Accessed May 7, 2025. https://www.law.cornell.edu/regulations/massachusetts/651-CMR-12-04

47. Kemp CL, Luo S, Ball MM. "Meds are a real tricky area": examining medication management and regulation in assisted living. J Appl Gerontol Off J South Gerontol Soc. 2012;31(1):126–49. https://doi.org/10.1177/0733464810381986.
48. Contributing Factors to Medication Nonadherence in an Assisted Living Facility. Accessed March 24, 2025. https://www.proquest.com/docview/1449137500?pq-origsite=gscholar&fromopenview=true&sourcetype=Dissertations%20&%20Theses
49. Zimmerman S, Guo W, Mao Y, Li Y, Temkin-Greener H. Health care needs in assisted living: survey data may underestimate chronic conditions. J Am Med Dir Assoc. 2021;22(2):471–3. https://doi.org/10.1016/j.jamda.2020.11.036.
50. Life Safety Code & Health Care Facilities Code (HCFC). Accessed March 24, 2025. https://www.cms.gov/medicare/health-safety-standards/guidance-for-laws-regulations/life-safety-code-health-care-facilities-code-hcfc
51. State Regulations for Assisted Living Facilities (All States). Accessed March 24, 2025. https://www.myfieldaudits.com/blog/state-regulations-for-assisted-living
52. Ohio Administrative Code. Rule 3701-16-15. Accessed March 24, 2025. https://codes.ohio.gov/ohio-administrative-code/rule-3701-16-15
53. Code of Federal Regulations. 42 CFR Part 483 - Requirements for States and Long-Term Care Facilities. Accessed March 24, 2025. https://www.ecfr.gov/current/title-42/part-483
54. Emergency Preparedness. Accessed March 24, 2025. https://www.ahcancal.org/Survey-Regulatory-Legal/Emergency-Preparedness/Pages/default.aspx
55. Abbasi J. COVID-19 crisis advances efforts to reimagine nursing homes. JAMA. 2021;326(16):1568–70. https://doi.org/10.1001/jama.2021.13326.
56. Nursing Homes Fought Federal Emergency Plan Requirements for Years. Now, They're Coronavirus Hot Spots. Accessed March 24, 2025. https://www.propublica.org/article/nursing-homes-fought-federal-emergency-plan-requirements-for-years-now-theyre-coronavirus-hot-spots
57. COVID-19: Critical Vaccine Distribution, Supply Chain, Program Integrity, and Other Challenges Require Focused Federal Attention. January 28, 2021. Accessed May 7, 2025. https://www.gao.gov/products/gao-21-265
58. Kaskie B, Xu L, Taylor S, et al. Promoting quality of life and safety in assisted living: a survey of state monitoring and enforcement agents. Med Care Res Rev. 2022;79(5):731–7. https://doi.org/10.1177/10775587211053410.
59. Temkin-Greener H, Guo W, Mao Y, Cai X, Li Y. COVID-19 pandemic in assisted living communities: results from seven states. J Am Geriatr Soc. 2020;68(12):2727–34. https://doi.org/10.1111/jgs.16850.
60. Guo W, Li Y, Temkin-Greener H. Coronavirus disease 2019 (COVID-19) in assisted living communities: neighborhood deprivation and state social distancing policies matter. Infect Control Hosp Epidemiol. 2022;43(8):1004–9. https://doi.org/10.1017/ice.2022.46.
61. Rep. Gray WH. H.R.3545 - 100th Congress (1987-1988): Omnibus budget reconciliation act of 1987. December 22, 1987. Accessed March 30, 2025. https://www.congress.gov/bill/100th-congress/house-bill/3545
62. Compendium of Residential Care and Assisted Living Regulations and Policy: 2015 Edition. https://aspe.hhs.gov/reports/compendium-residential-care-assisted-living-regulations-policy-2015-edition-0. Accessed June 14, 2025.
63. Long-Term Care Ombudsman. Accessed March 30, 2025. https://ohio.gov/residents/resources/office-of-the-state-long-term-care-ombudsman
64. Long-Term Care Ombudsman. Accessed March 30, 2025. https://aging.ca.gov/Programs_and_Services/Long-Term_Care_Ombudsman/
65. Missed Nursing Care: A Key Measure for Patient Safety. Accessed March 30, 2025. https://psnet.ahrq.gov/perspective/missed-nursing-care-key-measure-patient-safety
66. Ombudsman: Overview of Long-Term Care Ombudsman. Accessed March 30, 2025. https://www.in.gov/ombudsman/long-term-care-ombudsman/overview/
67. Massachusetts Long-Term Care Ombudsman Program. Accessed March 30, 2025. https://www.mass.gov/orgs/massachusetts-long-term-care-ombudsman-program

68. Long-Term Care Ombudsman. Accessed March 30, 2025. https://www.ncdhhs.gov/divisions/aging/long-term-care-ombudsman
69. Institute of Medicine (US) committee to evaluate the state long-term care ombudsman programs. Real people real problems: an evaluation of the long-term care ombudsman programs of the Older Americans Act. National Academies Press (US); 1995. Accessed March 30, 2025. http://www.ncbi.nlm.nih.gov/books/NBK231095/
70. Kemp CL, Ball MM, Morgan JC, et al. Exposing the backstage: critical reflections on a longitudinal qualitative study of residents' care networks in assisted living. Qual Health Res. 2017;27(8):1190–202. https://doi.org/10.1177/1049732316668817.
71. Moilanen T, Kangasniemi M, Papinaho O, et al. Older People's perceived autonomy in residential care: an integrative review. Nurs Ethics. 2021;28(3):414–34. https://doi.org/10.1177/0969733020948115.
72. Sikorska-Simmons E. The effects of organizational policies on resident perceptions of autonomy in assisted living. J Hous Elder. 2007;20(4):61–77. https://doi.org/10.1300/J081v20n04_05.
73. Harrington C, Mollot R, Braun RT, Williams D. United States' nursing home finances: spending, profitability, and capital structure. Int J Soc Determinants Health Health Serv. 2024;54(2):131–42. https://doi.org/10.1177/27551938231221509.
74. Werner RM, Konetzka RT. Reimagining financing and payment of long-term care. J Am Med Dir Assoc. 2022;23(2):220–4. https://doi.org/10.1016/j.jamda.2021.11.030.
75. Grabowski DC, Chen A, Saliba D. Paying for nursing home quality: an elusive but important goal. J Am Geriatr Soc. 2023;71(2):342–8. https://doi.org/10.1111/jgs.18260.
76. Silver BC, Grabowski DC, Gozalo PL, Dosa D, Thomas KS. Increasing prevalence of assisted living as a substitute for private-pay long-term nursing care. Health Serv Res. 2018;53(6):4906–20. https://doi.org/10.1111/1475-6773.13021.
77. Markowitz P. Hidden costs of assisted living care. Senior Living Specialists. Accessed March 30, 2025. https://www.seniorlivingspecialists.com/2024/03/hidden-costs-of-assisted-living-care/
78. All-Inclusive vs. A la Carte: Which Pricing Structure is Best for Assisted Living. Accessed May 8, 2025. https://arborsassistedliving.com/blog/all-inclusive-vs-a-la-carte-which-pricing-structure-is-best-for-assisted-living/
79. Pricing - Benton House. Accessed May 8, 2025. https://www.bentonhouse.com/pricing/
80. Caporaletti B. Pricing structure in assisted living. Accessed May 8, 2025. https://inglesideonline.org/blog/pricing-structure-in-assisted-living/
81. Understanding assisted living care pricing models. Accessed May 8, 2025. https://www.ambriantlife.com/post/understanding-assisted-living-care-pricing-models
82. Disclosures of Ownership and Additional Disclosable Parties Information for Skilled Nursing Facilities and Nursing Facilities. Accessed March 30, 2025. https://www.federalregister.gov/documents/2023/11/17/2023-25408/medicare-and-medicaid-programs-disclosures-of-ownership-and-additional-disclosable-parties
83. Weems J, Thomas K. Variation in state enforcement regulations regarding financial penalties against assisted living facilities. Innov Aging. 2022;6(Suppl 1):782. https://doi.org/10.1093/geroni/igac059.2828.
84. Thomas KS, Zhang W, Cornell PY, Smith L, Kaskie B, Carder PC. State variability in the prevalence and healthcare utilization of assisted living residents with dementia. J Am Geriatr Soc. 2020;68(7):1504–11. https://doi.org/10.1111/jgs.16410.
85. Mao Y, Li Y, McGarry B, Wang J, Temkin-Greener H. Home time and state regulations among Medicare beneficiaries in assisted living communities. J Am Geriatr Soc. 2024;72(3):742–52. https://doi.org/10.1111/jgs.18709.
86. Assisted Living Disclosure Collaborative: A National Initiative. Accessed March 30, 2025. https://www.theceal.org/information-2/projects-and-national-initiatives/2-uncategorised/14-assisted-living-disclosure-collaborative-a-national-initiative
87. A Study of Negotiated Risk Agreements in Assisted Living: Final Report. February 12, 2006. Accessed December 23, 2025. http://aspe.hhs.gov/reports/study-negotiated-risk-agreements-assisted-living-final-report-1

88. Belanger E, Rosendaal N, Wang XJ, et al. Association between state regulations supportive of third-party services and likelihood of assisted living residents in the US dying in place. JAMA Health Forum. 2022;3(10):e223432. https://doi.org/10.1001/jamahealthforum.2022.3432.

Chapter 4
The Assisted Living Workforce

Lindsay B. Schwartz

Introduction

In assisted living communities workforce plays a vital role providing *assistance,* focusing on residents' needs and preferences (i.e., person-centered care), and helping them to continue *living* in place for as long as possible [1]. The assistance the workforce provides varies greatly depending on state regulations and the assisted living organization [1]. To provide holistic, person-centered care the workforce needs comprehensive, on-going training to meet the medical and psychosocial needs of the residents. Ensuring employment opportunities are attractive, workers need to make a living wage, receive benefits, have opportunities for professional development, and other important supports. Without addressing these critical needs, staff will not be able to meet the needs of the residents and fulfill the promise of assistance and person-centered care. To fully understand the importance of the workforce to assisted living communities, it helps to examine who these workers are, staff composition, education and training, and the regulations that govern them.

Direct Care Professionals, Nurses, Physicians, and Social Workers

The COVID-19 pandemic revealed what many in long-term care industry already knew: direct care professionals (DCPs) are essential workers who provide care to our most vulnerable population [2,3]. There are some similarities between staff at assisted living, nursing homes, and other long-term care (LTC) settings. It is not unusual for staff to work at both assisted living communities and nursing homes, especially if they

L. B. Schwartz (✉)
Workforce & Quality Innovations, Bear Creek, NC, USA
e-mail: lindsay@wqinnovations.com

H. Temkin-Greener and S. Zimmerman (eds.), *Assisted Living Through Research, Policy, and Practice*, https://doi.org/10.1007/978-3-032-32088-9_4

work at a continuing care retirement community (CCRC) or for a company that owns or manages different levels of care. Due to federal regulations and higher resident acuity, there are more licensed clinical staff in nursing homes including registered nurses (RNs), licensed practical or vocational nurses (LPN/LVNs), and certified nursing aides (CNAs) to provide direct care. Some assisted living communities, depending on state regulations, have CNAs or certified medication aides (CMA). In these communities, DCPs may hold different titles depending on state regulations and the assisted living that employs them. In this chapter, we use the term DCPs which include personal care aides, universal workers (who do other tasks including food service and housekeeping), aides, CNAs, CMAs, and other titles used in assisted living for individuals providing direct care to residents.

There are 455,900 nursing and social work full time equivalent (FTE) employees in assisted living; this estimate includes DCPs which make up 75.4% of the total workforce [4]. These direct care professionals are mostly women (84%), over half (61%) are people of color, and 24% are immigrants [2]. They range in age between 16 and 65+ years, with a median of 40 [2]. Fifty-one percent of DCPs have some education past high school, including 20% who have an associate's or higher degree [2]. Salaries of direct care professionals are typically low, and they receive few, if any, employee benefits such as health insurance or paid time off (sick-time and vacation).[2] Some DCPs experience unstable employment, almost a fifth are employed only part of the year and 28% are part-time (35 hours a week or less) [2]. Many DCPs experience economic hardships, sixty-four percent live in low-income households (<200% of the federal poverty level) and of these, 11% are below the federal poverty level [2]. Thirty-five percent of DCPs are on Medicaid or other government health insurance coverage and may receive other assistance including supplemental nutrition assistance program (SNAP) [2]. These hardships may impact the DCP's ability to be successful in their occupation.

Direct care professionals provide most of the care in assisted living, which includes assistance with activities of daily living (ADLs) and instrumental activities of daily living (IADLs) [6]. The work requires an array of skills from caregiving and communication, infection prevention, health literacy, emotional intelligence, relational and problem-solving skills. Still, DCPs are at times referred to as "low-skilled" or "unskilled" which is not only inaccurate but also demeaning to these essential workers [2,3,5,6]. These professionals spend roughly 4 hours per resident per day (3.8) in direct care, the highest of the nursing and social work professions [4]. Since DCPs spend so much time with residents, they typically know them well and they play an important role in the care team; a recent assisted living expert panel study recommended that DCPs should be part of the assessment/care planning team [9]. The DCPs also provide social and emotional support to assisted living residents, which is important to quality of life and health outcomes [10]. Typically, DCPs supplement this type of support provided by residents' family and friends, but during the COVID-19 pandemic, residents experienced significant declines of in-person visits, due in part to state or assisted living community restrictions on visitors [11]. While DCPs are not licensed, except for CNAs and CMAs, some states have certifications for direct care workers, for example Wisconsin's Certified Direct Care Professional (CDCP) program [12].

Thirty-seven states and the District of Columbia require that RN or LPN/LVN provide or supervise care in assisted living or be available as needed [13–15]. The nurses can be directly employed or contracted [14]. Several states allow residents with higher acuity to remain in assisted living, by allowing nurses to practice to their full license or a third party (e.g., hospice or home health) to provide the skilled care [13–15]. Nurses provide critical services that include resident assessments both initially and when a change in condition occurs, or at regularly scheduled or required intervals (e.g., 90 days, 120 days, annually) [13–15]. Nurses may distribute, administer, or oversee the administration of medications (both orally and by injection), though in some states staff may only be allowed to support residents as they self-medicate, and others allow CMAs, CNAs, or other unlicensed staff who are trained to administer medications [13–15]. Depending on state regulations, nurses may be allowed to check residents' blood sugar and other vitals including oxygen level and blood pressure. Nurses may administer vaccinations to both residents and staff. One study, based on 455 assisted living communities in Ohio, found that increases in RN hours were associated with reduced injury-related emergency department visits, but not with hospital admissions for residents with Alzheimer's disease or related dementias (ADRD) [16].

The National Center for Health Statistics (NCHS) 2022 National Post-Acute and Long-Term Care Study (NPALS) estimated RNs provided 0.5 hours per resident per day and LPN/LVNs 0.4 hours per resident per day in residential care communities (RCC) that employed nurses [4]. The NPALS uses the term RCCs as inclusive of assisted living and other terminology states use to define these communities. It is important to note that this study included RCCs that did not have nurses on staff. For the 2022 NPALS survey, NCHS used lists of licensed RCCs in each state and the District of Columbia (DC) which resulted in a sampling frame of 46,049 RCCs [17] A random sample of 2088 RCCs was selected and of the eligible RCCs, 688 completed the provider survey [17]. To account for the smaller sample, NCHS used weights to ensure the data are representative of assisted-living communities.[17]

Physicians (MDs, DOs), physician assistants (PAs), and nurse practitioners (NPs) are also integral to the resident care teams in assisted living communities, whether they are employees or contract staff [8,13–15]. A panel of experts highly recommend assisted living communities to have a medical care provider on-site [9]. Typically larger communities or chains have a Chief Medical Officer and Medical Directors overseeing the care of the residents [15] Smaller or independently owned communities may contract with a Medical Director that oversees a number of other assisted living communities. An innovation that some communities have implemented is having a walk-in clinic on-site for residents, staff, and family members of residents and staff. This has enabled the assisted living communities to have an MD/DO, PA, or NP available more often. Most assisted living does not have a full-time social worker and instead contract or have one available part-time.

Dining, Housekeeping, Administrative, and Other Staff

Presence of other staff depends on the assisted living size, whether it is part of a chain, a regional organization in multiple states, or independently owned. Typically, all communities have housekeeping staff that do laundry, clean main areas and residents' apartments. Dining and food preparation staff include chefs, cooks, and dining aides or wait staff. Both housekeeping and dining staff get to know the residents well as they have a lot of interaction with them and find out their preferences for food, who their friends are, and how they like their apartment kept.

Larger assisted living providing services in multiple states typically have a main office with leadership and support staff. Many assisted living organizations have administrative staff including marketing, human resources, and billing. Administrative staff may be at a regional or main office or co-located within the community, depending on the size of the company. In smaller and independently owned communities, the Executive Director (Administrator) or owner may wear many hats and fill multiple roles on the team. Contractors may be hired in place of staff for maintenance, housekeeping, human resources, or laundry service. Activity directors plan parties and activity programs for residents with assistance from activity aides or DCPs. This is an important role, as assisted living is known for social activities including outings, bringing in musicians, screening movies, and other events. For outings, shopping, and doctor's appointments, most assisted living communities offer a van or shuttle.

Family, Friends, and Volunteers

Employees of assisted living communities are not the only important team members; family, friends, and volunteers also serve a critical role, at times providing or supplementing the care residents receive. The importance of these individuals was apparent during the COVID-19 pandemic, when many states and LTC providers banned visitors to try and keep residents from contracting the virus. Some states allowed family, friends, and volunteers to be in assisted living as essential caregivers, requiring them to follow the same precautions as staff (vaccination, masks, social distancing, etc.) [8,18].

State Workforce Regulations

Staffing, Oversight, and Licensing

State regulations typically dictate basic required staffing patterns and ratios in assisted living. Nineteen states have minimum staffing ratios but vary as to the degree of specificity [19,20]. Some state regulations require "sufficient" number of staff without specifying details [19,20]. Most staffing ratios are for DCPs and nurses [19,20]. In 2021, the Oregon Senate passed a bill to develop and assess an acuity-based staffing tool for DCPs [21]. A panel of nineteen assisted living experts agreed a DCP-to-resident staffing ratio was important and should be based on resident acuity [9]

Research has demonstrated the importance of the state DCP regulatory specificity for resident outcomes. For example, higher staffing specificity for DCPs was shown to be associated with a decrease in residents' hospital admissions [23].

State Training Requirements

Initial and on-going training for staff is critical to ensure residents receive person-centered, high-quality care. Regardless of who provides the training, the employer should have documentation and verification of training completion that employees receive and can take to another job, if they leave [24]. Staff should at least receive training upon hire and annually, but at a minimum as required by state regulations. Training should cover the basics of caring for an individual and other topics for staff to excel in their profession. Initial and on-going training requirements, including the number of hours of training for administrators and DCPs, vary widely across states [1]. All but three states require initial training for DCPs, but most do not specify how much training or its content [3]. Forty-four states require on-going training for both administrators and DCPs. Thirty-three states require training for DCPs but do not specify the number of hours and nineteen states specify the number of hours required [19]. Assisted living providers may have additional training requirements for staff including disease-specific training.

Residents who passed away in assisted living communities located in states with greater specificity in training requirements had significantly fewer end-of-life care transfers compared to communities in other states [25].

Even though states and licensing organizations have specific training requirements for staff with degrees and licenses, it is still important that all staff are trained on topics specific to the community and residents. The focus of most training in assisted living is how to care for residents (assisting with activities of daily living (ADLs) and instrumental activities of daily living (IADLs)), but additional training can benefit both residents and staff. A panel of experts rated the following training topics as high importance for assisted living staff: person-centered care, dementia and mental illness, side effects of medication (for staff who administer medication), infection prevention and control, end-of-life care and advance care planning [9]. The Assisted Living Workgroup (ALW) included staff training in many of their recommendations in the 2003 report to the U.S. Senate Special Committee on Aging [18].

Federal Workforce Regulations and Guidance

Even though assisted living is regulated at the state level, there are federal regulations that apply to the assisted living workforce and their employers. Depending on the regulation, some employers are exempt or partially exempt depending on the number of employees. For example, in the OSHA Standard 1904.1, the Recording and Reporting Occupational Injuries and Illnesses, employers with 10 or less employees are exempt from reporting injuries and illnesses but not exempt from reporting fatalities to OSHA [27].

Workforce Challenges and Recommendations

Workforce is one of the top concerns for assisted living providers, including staff burnout, turnover, recruitment, and supply of trained workers [29]. There are not a lot of evidence-based solutions on recruiting and retaining assisted living staff [22].

Recruitment, Retention, Turnover, and Quality Care Jobs

Assisted living providers have used numerous tactics to recruit staff. From using job boards, attending career fairs, or posting positions online, to sponsoring a local kids' baseball team, advertising on the assisted living shuttle or van, and letting residents and families know the assisted living is hiring.

The Gerontological Society of America (GSA) created Careers in Aging Week (CIAW). During this week, GSA hosted activities for members of GSA to talk about their careers to engage potential workers to the field. After a number of years of success with CIAW, GSA welcomed trade associations that represent assisted living and nursing homes to participate and expand the reach of Careers in Aging to celebrate current LTC staff and recruit staff. This initiative has expanded from a week to a month and includes additional organizations. Oregon Care Careers developed a website that provides education, training, and job duties of the different roles in LTC and potential career paths [30]. Job seekers can also work with a career navigator who can share potential careers in LTC and what training they would need [30]. The site includes job postings and a link to Oregon Care Partners that provides free training [30].

COVID-19 turned a workforce shortage into a crisis due to burnout, safety concerns, and emotional exhaustion [8,31]. Leadership and DCPs in assisted living identified different factors that led to turnover during COVID-19. Direct care professionals attributed turnover to low pay, high ratios of residents to staff, and lack of recognition [31]. Nurses and DCPs reported feeling "overwhelmed" due to staffing shortages [31]. They reported feeling "undervalued" and "unsupported" [31]. Staff were not able to access services like online therapy due to staffing shortages [31].

Assisted living leadership attributed turnover to external issues such as state policies and systemic issues including the demanding work of direct care [31].

Research has found that factors predicting staff retention in nursing homes also predict retention of staff in assisted living, where retention levels are higher [22]. Assisted living communities are more likely to use consistent assignment and provide cross training, both of which may lead to higher staff retention [22]. Including DCPs in resident care planning is also thought to be linked to higher retention rates [9,22].

Providing care is a hard job for which staff deserve fair compensation, including access to full time hours, a living wage, employer, or union-sponsored benefit plans, paid sick and vacation days, family medical leave (FMLA), grief support, and bereavement leave [8,18,24]. Assisted living providers need to be competitive with pay and benefits or staff will go elsewhere. When recruiting potential employees, assisted living employers need to share information about the entire benefit package, not just salary and do this annually, during benefit election time. Benefit packages can include health insurance, retirement contributions or matches, short and long-term disability, life insurance, gym memberships, professional development opportunities, money for continuing education or conference attendance.

Employers should be clear on job requirements, responsibilities, workflows, and reporting structures [18,24]. This information should be available in print and posted in a staff shared space, e.g., a breakroom. All staff should have consistent, accessible, and supportive supervision [24]. Frequent employee turnover usually reflects poor organizational practices and management [33]. One way of supporting employees is through peer mentoring programs and support networks [24]. Such programs can lead to higher productivity, better pay and promotions, and lower turnover [24].

A safe and supportive environment is important to both staff and residents. Research has shown that in assisted living communities, perceptions of work environment quality are different for DCPs and for administrators, with the former viewing safety culture within their organizations as being worse compared to the latter [34]. Both administrators and DCPs reported communication openness, non-punitive response, management support and teamwork as domains important to safety culture in assisted living [34].

Similarly, research suggests that physical environment for employees working in LTC may reduce or exacerbate workforce burnout and attrition. Recent studies identified several specific space types and design characteristics, relevant to LTC work environments, that were deemed supportive of employee health and well-being [35]. Such space design recommendations, although less common, may include providing outdoor break space, a restorative space/room, a lactation room, fitness room or space, shower facilities, secured storage space or lockers [35].

Implications for "Assisted" and "Living"

In assisted living, a stable workforce is the most essential element in ensuring the residents are appropriately *assisted* and the quality of their *living* is promoted. Today, many assisted living communities struggle as they try providing person-centered care and meeting many of the medical and psychosocial needs of their residents. With rising resident acuity, the assisted living workforce needs to be continuously well-trained to assist residents and "promote their quality of living" [6]. To be able to meet these needs, assisted living communities need to have the right staff including clinical staff. Direct care professionals and other staff need on-going training that includes learning about each resident so they can truly provide person-centered care. To accomplish this, assisted living providers need to offer good jobs that maximize staff retention and minimize turnover. With the staffing shortages in the LTC sector, assisted living employers need to refocus on better staff recruitment and retainment initiatives.

State regulations which govern staffing and training of assisted living workforce may either facilitate or hinder residents' receipt of sufficient and appropriate *assistance* that addresses their care needs and facilitate continued *living* in the community. However, regulations do not entirely drive practice, as evident in communities where workforce is sufficient, and staff are well trained in supporting and allowing residents to age in place.

Workforce challenges are multi-faceted and thus require a multi-prong approach that requires providers, policymakers, employees, and family members of the residents to ensure that assisted living keeps its promise of sufficient *assistance* to support residents *living* as independently as possible with good quality of life.

Competing Interests The author has no conflicts of interest to declare that are relevant to the content of this chapter.

References

1. Zimmerman S, Carder P, Schwartz L, Silbersack J, Temkin-Greener H, et al. The imperative to reimagine assisted living. J Am Med Dir Assoc. 2022;23(2):225–34.
2. Scales K, Lepore MJ. Always essential: valuing direct care workers in long-term care. Public Policy Aging Rep. 2020;
3. Drake A. Direct care work is real work: elevating the role of the direct care worker. PHI; 2020.
4. National Post Acute and Long-Term Care Study [Internet] Table 2: Staffing characteristics of post-acute and long-term care providers: United States. 2020. Available from: https://www.cdc.gov/nchs/npals/webtables/overview.htm
5. PHI. Direct care workers in the United States: Key facts 2024.
6. Zimmerman S, Stone R, Carder P, Thomas K. Does assisted living provide assistance and promote living? Health Aff. 2024;43(5):674–81.
7. Tyler DA, Khavjou O, Hunter M, Kristie P, Horvath M, Suarez G, Squillace MR, Dey J. State efforts to improve direct care workforce wages: Final report. Assistant Secretary for Planning and Evaluation at the U.S. Department of Health & Human Services; 2024 January 9, 2024.

8. Schwartz LB, Lieblich C, Laxton CE, Kaes L, Barnett DP, Port C, Pace DD. COVID-19 in assisted living: protecting a critical long-term care resource. J Am Med Dir Assoc. 2023;
9. Zimmerman S, Sloane PD, Wretman CJ, Cao K, Silbersack J, Carder P, Thomas KS, Allen J, Butrum K, Chicotel T, Giorgio P, Hernandez M, Kales H, Katz P, Klinger JH, Kunze M, Laxton C, McNealley V, Meeks S, O'Neil K, Pace DD, Resnick B, Schwartz LB, Seitz D, Smetanka L, Van Haitsma K. Recommendations for medical and mental health care in assisted living based on an expert Delphi consensus panel: a consensus statement. JAMA Netw Open. 2022;5(9)
10. Academies N, of Sciences, Engineering, and Medicine. Social isolation and loneliness in older adults: opportunities for the health care system. Washington, DC: The National Academies Press; 2020.
11. Freedman VA, Hu M, Kasper JD. Changes in older adults' social contact during the COVID-19 pandemic. J Gerontol B Psychol Sci Soc Sci. 2021;77(7):e160–e6.
12. Wisconsin Department of Health Services and University of Wisconsin Green Bay. WisCaregiver Careers: Certified Direct Care Professional. 2023. Available from: https://www.dhs.wisconsin.gov/library/collection/p-03346
13. Beeber AS, Zimmerman S, Madeline Mitchell C, Reed D. Staffing and service availability in assisted living: the importance of nurse delegation policies. J Am Geriatr Soc. 2018;66(11):2158–66.
14. Rome V, Harris-Kojetin L, Carder P. Variation in licensed nurse staffing characteristics by state requirements in residential care. Res Gerontol Nurs. 2019;12(1):27–33.
15. Dys S, Smith L, Tunalilar O, Carder P. Revisiting the role of physicians in assisted living and tesidential care settings. Gerontol Geriatr Med. 2020;6:2333721420979840.
16. Hua CL, Nelson I, Cornell PY, White EM, Thomas KS. Changes in nursing staff levels and injury-related emergency department visits among assisted living residents with Alzheimers disease and related dementias. J Am Med Dir Assoc. 2024;25(8):105087.
17. National Center for Health Statistics. 2022 National post-acute and long-term care study survey methodology for the adult day services center and residential care community components. Centers for Disease Control; 2022.
18. Assisted Living Workgroup. Assuring quality in assisted living: guidelines for federal and state policy, state regulations, and operations. Senate Special Committee on Aging: A report to the U.S; 2003.
19. Carder P, O'Keefe J, O'Keefe C, White E, Wiener JM. State regulatory provisions for residential care settings: an overview of staffing requirements. Research Triangle Park, NC. 2016; Publication No. OP-0030-1607
20. Temkin-Greener H, Mao Y, Ladwig S, Cai X, Zimmerman S, Li Y. Variability and potential determinants of assisted living state regulatory stringency. J Am Med Dir Assoc. 2021;22(8):1714–9.
21. Oregon department of human services. Acuity-based staffing overview 2025. Available from: https://www.oregon.gov/odhs/licensing/community-based-care/pages/acuity-based-staffing.aspx
22. Kennedy KA, Applebaum R, Bowblis JR, Straker JK. Organizational factors associated with retention of direct care workers: a comparison of nursing homes and assisted living facilities. Gerontologist. 2021;61(4):530–9.
23. Thomas KS, Cornell PY, Zhang W, Smith L, Hua C, Kaskie B, Carder P. The relationship between states' staffing regulations and hospitalizations of assisted living residents. Health Aff. 2021;40(9):1377–85.
24. PHI. The 5 Pillars of Direct Care Job Quality. 2020.
25. Guo W, Cai S, Caprio T, Schwartz L, Temkin-Greener H. End-of-life care transitions in assisted living: associations with state staffing and training regulations. J Am Med Dir Assoc. 2023;24(6):827–32.
26. Oregon Care Partners. About Oregon Care Partners. 2025. Available from: https://www.oregon.gov/odhs/licensing/community-based-care/pages/acuity-based-staffing.aspx
27. Occupational Safety and Health Administration. Recording and reporting occupational injuries and illnesses: Partial exemption for employers with 10 or fewer employees. Available from https://www.osha.gov/laws-regs/regulations/standardnumber/1904/1904.1.

28. Carder P, Dys S, Schwartz LB, Jacoby D, Kohon J, Himes D, Fox M, Elliot S, Bouchard L. Direct care staff experiences in Oregon assisted living, residential care and memory care communities, 2022. Portland, OR: Portland State University Institute on Aging; 2023.
29. Oregon Care Careers. 2025. Available from: https://oregoncarecareers.com/.
30. Yuan Y. Navigating high staff turnover: how organizational hierarchy shaped assisted living facility employees' emotional responses during the COVID-19 pandemic. Socius. 2025;11:23780231251350173.
31. Wiener JM, Elkins W, Lepore MJ. Impacts of potential minimum wage increases on assisted living and continuing care retirement communities. RTI International and Center for Excellence in Assisted Living (CEAL); 2017.
32. Brannon D, Barry T, Kemper P, Schreiner A, Vasey J. Job perceptions and intent to leave among direct care workers: evidence from the better jobs better care demonstrations. Gerontologist. 2007;47(6):820–9.
33. Temkin-Greener H, Mao Y, McGarry B, Zimmerman S. Patient safety culture in assisted living: staff perceptions and association with state regulations. J Am Med Dir Assoc. 2022;23(12):1997–02.
34. Goldman CM, Rider TR, Fisher GG, Loder AL, Schwatka NV, Van Dyke MV. Designing LTC physical work environments to support worker Well-being: a review and recommendations. J Am Med Dir Assoc. 2025;26(1)
35. Mercurio Z. The power of mattering at work. Harv Bus Rev. 2025;

Chapter 5
Dementia and Dementia Care in Assisted Living

Philip D. Sloane, Sheryl Zimmerman, David Balter, and Elizabeth Morton

Introduction

Because persons living with dementia typically require supportive rather than medical care, assisted living (AL) communities have surpassed nursing homes to become the primary residential long-term care setting for older adults living with dementia. In response to this demographic shift, the prevalence, needs, and care of persons with dementia in AL has become the focus of research, policy, and practice [1], and controversial issues have come to light that remain unresolved. This chapter summarizes data on the demography of dementia in AL and related needs and care planning and discusses some key contentious issues that remain unresolved.

P. D. Sloane (✉)
Department of Family Medicine, School of Medicine; Program On Aging, Chronic Illness, and Long-Term Care; and the Cecil G. Sheps Center for Health Services Research, University of North Carolina at Chapel Hill, Chapel Hill, NC, USA
e-mail: philip_sloane@med.unc.edu

S. Zimmerman
Center for Excellence in Assisted Living (CEAL@UNC), School of Social Work and the Cecil G. Sheps Center for Health Services Research, University of North Carolina at Chapel Hill, Chapel Hill, NC, USA
e-mail: Sheryl_Zimmerman@unc.edu

D. Balter
School of Social Work, University of North Carolina at Chapel Hill, Chapel Hill, NC, USA
e-mail: dbalter@unc.edu

E. Morton
School of Medicine, University of North Carolina at Chapel Hill, Chapel Hill, NC, USA
e-mail: Elizabeth_Morton@med.unc.edu

H. Temkin-Greener and S. Zimmerman (eds.), *Assisted Living Through Research, Policy, and Practice*, https://doi.org/10.1007/978-3-032-32088-9_5

Identifying, Diagnosing, and Assessing Cognitive Impairment, Dementia, and Alzheimer's Disease

Cognition refers to a wide range of mental functions of varying complexity, and terms referring to cognitive impairment are not applied universally. For example, neurologists, geriatricians, and much of the general public use the term "dementia" to describe conditions characterized by severe cognitive loss, and "mild cognitive impairment" to describe less severe impairment. Psychiatrists prefer the terms "major neurocognitive disorder" and "mild neurocognitive disorder" to describe the same conditions [2, 3]. Because the terms cognitive impairment and dementia are more common, they are used in this chapter.

In most cognitive disorders of aging, including Alzheimer's disease, the more complex functions tend to become impaired earlier, and gradually, over years, other functions become affected.

- High-level cognitive function tends to be lost early in cognitive disorders (i.e., in mild cognitive impairment). These functions include such things as planning, learning new ideas, organization, and recent or complex memory. Managing a household, including financial matters, requires these skills, which explains why many individuals entering AL have mild cognitive impairment. Behavioral expressions, such as repeated questioning, mood changes, and anxiety, are also common in mild cognitive disorders.
- As cognitive loss advances into dementia, memory loss is more severe, and physical function becomes impaired. A common strategy to assess advancing impairment is to determine whether the individual can independently conduct various activities of daily living (ADLs); of these, bathing, dressing, and grooming are often the first to need assistance. As dementia progresses, more functions are affected, including the ability to walk, use the toilet, and eventually to eat and turn over in bed. Loss of language parallels these declines, such that people with advanced dementia generally have limited verbal skills. Behavioral expressions are present as well and often change as physical abilities and care requirements change—for example, wandering ceases to be a problem when the ability to ambulate becomes impaired, but pain and anxiety-related behavioral expressions such as hitting or yelling become more common with increased cognitive impairment.

That said, variation exists in the trajectory and pattern of cognitive loss depending on the individual and diagnosis. The four most common dementia diagnoses in older persons residing in AL are described briefly below [4, 5].

- **Alzheimer's disease** is the most common dementia diagnosis. Slowly progressive memory loss is prominent, accompanied by gradual impairment of first high-level and then more basic cognitive functions. Behavioral expressions are common and vary markedly from person to person.
- **Vascular dementia** is also common, caused by problems in circulation to the brain. It has a variety of forms but classically is differentiated from Alzheimer's disease in that progression tends to be stepwise, with periods of stability followed

by rapid decline, presumably from a new stroke. In addition, vascular injury within the brain tends to be spotty rather than uniform, and people with vascular dementia will often have relatively preserved areas of memory or speech even when the disease is advanced.

- **Frontotemporal dementia** is a group of syndromes characterized by early age of onset, and by early and marked changes in personality, emotion, and impulse control. Other symptoms that can be prominent include inertia, loss of empathy, changes in food preferences and eating habits, and in one variant, early loss of word finding and verbal expression as well as gradual memory loss.
- **Dementia with Lewy bodies** (DLB) is also quite common. In addition to memory loss and behavioral changes, persons with DLB tend to have features much like those of persons with Parkinson's disease, such as resting tremor, shuffling gait, hallucinations, and disordered sleep.

However, diagnostic clarity is complicated because many people with cognitive impairment have more than one dementia diagnosis, most commonly with vascular disease being a secondary factor. In addition, cognitive impairment from neurological disease can be compounded by the effects of medications and chronic diseases such as heart failure. From a care perspective, the exact cause of cognitive impairment may be relatively unimportant because the principles of management are largely the same regardless of the diagnosis. What is more important is identifying that cognitive impairment is present, determining its severity and main characteristics, and developing an individualized care and service plan [6].

The Increasing Prevalence of Residents with Dementia in Assisted Living

In 2022, 44% of AL residents had a diagnosis of dementia [7]. Dementia prevalence varied by community size, with smaller communities tending to have higher proportions of persons with dementia—51% in communities with 4–25 beds compared to 39% in communities with more than 50 beds [1, 8]. These numbers were a marked increase from 1992, when 28% of AL residents had dementia [9], reflecting an overall rise in dementia diagnoses by the medical community [10], increased focus on dementia services by AL providers [11], and appeal to family members because of the perception that AL is more person-centered than nursing homes [11, 12].

Furthermore, as the proportion of AL residents with a diagnosis of dementia approaches 50%, many more may have undiagnosed dementia, as over 70% of AL residents have some form of cognitive impairment [1]. Indeed, one study involving careful neuropsychiatric assessment found that 38% of AL residents without a diagnosis of dementia had probable dementia and an additional 52% had mild cognitive impairment [13]. Knowing that dementia is underdiagnosed, AL communities are advised to screen the cognitive status of all residents on admission and periodically during re-evaluation to inform care and service needs [13].

Persons with dementia generally enter AL because they are unable to live independently and have exceeded the capacity of their families to provide the support needed to remain at home. On average, AL residents with dementia have impairment in 2 of 5 basic activities of daily living, most commonly bathing [1]. Among the challenges that often accompany dementia are impaired vision and/or hearing; impaired judgment, problem-solving, planning, organizational skills, and communication; and certain behavioral expressions, such as agitation and aggression, all of which can interfere with the individual's ability to live independently [14].Another significant challenge for people with dementia is an increased risk of falls due to a combination of frailty, impaired decision-making, and sensitivity to many medications [15].

Assisted Living in the Context of Other Residential Care Options for Persons with Dementia

The care offered by AL communities aims to assist with activities of daily living while providing a homelike environment; communities that expressly serve people living with dementia generally have safety measures in place, such as exit monitoring/control and handrails in hallways and bathrooms [16]. They also have activity programming that strives to engage residents and help them remain socially engaged, and they ideally offer access to the outdoors, ranging from a patio or garden to excursions into the community [16, 17].

In general, AL follows a model of care that focuses more on psychosocial and supportive needs rather than medical and ongoing nursing needs, and the communities market themselves as embracing a person-centered care philosophy and environment [16, 18]. Consequently, if the need for ongoing medical care arises, transfer to a nursing home may ensue; in fact, AL residents are hospitalized more frequently than nursing home residents, underscoring the point that AL is comparatively less equipped to handle medical care needs [19].

Some AL communities have developed specialized program or units for persons with dementia, but these are not the norm, and research has led to mixed results about their benefit. Across the country, about 20% of AL communities provide specialized memory care [20]. They tend to be larger, offer more services, and provide more medical care than communities that do not offer a dementia care program [21]. More detail on these programs is presented later in this chapter.

As the prevalence of cognitive impairment has increased over time, so too has overall medical acuity, which has led to an increased presence of licensed nurses in AL to aid in tasks such as medication administration, physical and cognitive assessment, and tube feeding [22, 23]. For persons who are deteriorating rapidly and prefer to remain in place, many AL communities offer hospice care through contracts with community agencies [24, 25]. All told, though, while AL may offer advantages to persons with dementia who do not need ongoing medical care, evidence is lacking to determine the best settings and characteristics of settings for residential long-term care of people with dementia [26].

Care Needs of Residents with Dementia

The care needs of AL residents with dementia are no different than the care needs of all persons living with dementia. They can be grouped hierarchically into five categories: [27]

- **Physiological needs**, such as physical comfort, nutrition, hydration, and sleep; personal hygiene; access to sunlight and fresh air; preservation of skin integrity; and management of symptoms such as pain, constipation, and shortness of breath.
- **Safety and security**, including safeguard of personal possessions; prevention and treatment of injury and illness; opportunity for privacy; and freedom from noxious stimuli such as noise, glare, and odor.
- **Social engagement**, including companionship, affection, touch, and family and friend visits; inclusion in the community; support of sexual expression; and, when needed, ameliorating sensory impairments such as vision and hearing loss to facilitate participation in social interactions.
- **Self-esteem**, including support for personal preferences, autonomy, dignity, and self-expression; environmental features that aid functional competence; and access to activities that are meaningful to the individual and that help maintain identity.
- **Optimal quality of life**, including such things as participation in expressive, creative, and spiritual activities; provision of ongoing opportunities for stimulation and rehabilitation; minimization of displeasure, anxiety, or boredom; and opportunity for life review and creation of legacy.

Beyond these universal needs, care for persons with dementia includes additional considerations related to environmental design for safety, wayfinding, and cueing; activity programs and approaches especially designed for persons with cognitive impairment; person-centered care practices that minimize confusion and avoid triggering agitation and other expressions of discomfort; and policies that embody and reinforce principles of person-centered dementia care. Each of these is described below.

Environmental design. The built environment is especially important in dementia because it can improve function by helping compensate for some deficits associated with cognitive loss. For example, to avoid confusion from not remembering the location of living and dining spaces, one aspect of dementia-friendly design involves small clusters in which bedrooms open directly into common areas [28]; another design feature makes the toilet visible from a resident's bed, thereby reducing incontinence episodes [29]. To maximize safety, exits can be disguised; gardens can be restricted to plants that are edible; and sturdy furniture and handrails can be positioned at key locations such as the pathway from the bed to the bathroom so as to reduce falls [30]. The environment can also function as a treatment; for example, bright light in the morning can improve night-time sleep, and reduction of noxious noises such as alarms can reduce anxiety [26].

Activities. Persons with dementia often have trouble initiating and doing things on their own, such as reading a newspaper, completing a jigsaw puzzle, or engaging in exercise; therefore, organized activities are especially important for persons with dementia. In AL, most residents with dementia retain the ability to understand simple statements, questions, and directions, and can socialize with others around them [31], indicating that the task for AL communities is to design and lead engaging activities that promote health, well-being, and quality of life [32]. Familiar activities are particularly useful, such as participation in meal preparation, laundry, and gardening, and adhering to a daily schedule [16].

Person-centered care. Most AL residents with dementia need support with daily functions such as bathing, dressing, and grooming. Because these encounters are among the most frequent interactions between AL staff and residents, they constitute a primary opportunity to enhance quality of life. Person-centered care includes focusing on and upholding the value of the person, being unhurried, having flexible approaches, and encouraging the resident to direct their care to the extent possible [33]. Person-centeredness extends to family visitors as well, by helping them develop meaningful roles within the care setting [34].

Dementia-aware policies. To reinforce dementia-appropriate environmental design, foster engaging activity programs, and promote person-centered care practices, it is recommended that AL communities have policies that embody dementia-awareness. Goals underlying these policies include: a familiar, pleasant atmosphere; resident well-being; a sense of belonging; individualized care; and meaningful relationships among residents, between residents and staff, among staff, and with families [32]. Policies are reinforced by supervisors and through regular training, such as educating staff to identify early signs of anxiety and discomfort and in response to change their care approach to promote resident comfort and quality of life [35].

Fostering Engagement and Positive Experiences

Engaging in meaningful activity is important to quality of life, but the promotion of meaningful engagement can be complicated by dementia. Common features of meaningful engagement include participation in activities consistent with interests and previous roles, and that promote identity, belonging, physical health, and independence [36–39]. Meaningful engagement is considered central to quality of life and high-quality, person-centered care [40–43].

Unfortunately, meaningful engagement is frequently an unmet need for people with dementia residing in AL and other forms of long-term care. Available activities are often inappropriate or inaccessible, and participation rates are consistently low [44, 45]. One study found that 45% of residents with dementia were provided limited or no activities, 20% were provided occasional activities, and 12% were provided daily activities that were inappropriate based on interests or functional level [46]. An example of an activity considered inappropriate is programming designed to entertain and distract rather than meaningfully engage residents, thus promoting isolated, sedentary behavior that may contribute to physical deconditioning, loneliness, and depression [44].

Of course, cognitive impairment poses challenges to effective engagement, as residents with dementia typically require increased assistance to engage with others [45, 47]; unfortunately, the need for more assistance is at times in juxtaposition to limitations in terms of staffing, staff training, resources, and care philosophy [17, 41, 48]. More specifically, high staff turnover is common in AL and may result in decreased opportunities for engagement when programming is canceled due to staff departures [41]. Also, limited understanding about dementia can negatively impact opportunities for engagement by fostering a belief that people with dementia are incapable of purposeful and meaningful communication and interaction, whereas what they actually need are structured and personalized opportunities for social inclusion and meaningful engagement [44, 49].

AL communities can best promote meaningful engagement for residents with dementia by employing basic dementia care approaches [41, 47, 50]:

- know the person, including their preferences and life history;
- connect with and meet the person where they are, such as by joining in their reality rather than correcting or arguing;
- be in the moment by remaining attentive and adapting to moods, situations, responses, and opportunities; and
- consider all encounters an opportunity for meaningful engagement, most notably support with activities of daily living.

Implementing these four strategies when caring for persons with dementia increases positive expressions such as smiling, concentration, and laughter, and decreases negative responses such as anxiety, anger, and frustration [47]. In addition, it is important to attend to residents' capacity for engagement, which is affected by their physical and cognitive function, care needs, motivation, energy, attention, and pain level [41]. Toward that end, additional recommendations include following the Alzheimer's Association's three care goals for meaningful activity and social engagement [40]:

- offer multiple opportunities daily that provide a sense of community, personal meaning, choice, and fun;
- create interactions "to do *with*, not *to* or *for*," the resident; and
- respect resident preferences, even if they prefer solitude.

More recently, a growing body of evidence supports the potential usefulness of technology—such as involvement through robotic pets and reminiscence through computer programming—to increase engagement among residents with dementia. However, engagement with technology must be thoughtful, applied in a person-centered manner, adapted to individual preferences, and promote human-to-human interaction, as opposed to merely being provided to residents without support and guidance; that said, more research is needed in this area, including to understand the perspective of people living with dementia regarding their experience with technology [51].

Understanding and Addressing Behavioral Expressions

Persons with dementia are often unable to convey the cause of discomfort or distress, and instead convey them with what has been widely referred to as "behavioral and psychological symptoms of dementia" (BPSDs) but are now better recognized as behavioral expressions of discomfort and distress [52]. Among behavioral expressions, agitation and aggression are especially common, occurring in 40–60% of people living with dementia [53, 54]. Additionally, dementia is a noted risk factor for residents' verbal, physical, and sexual aggression in AL [55]. Differentiating between agitation and aggression may help clarify how to properly predict and detect their occurrence. The International Psychogeriatric Association defines *agitation* as a syndrome that involves excessive motor or verbal activity [54]. *Aggression* is any verbal or physical behavior, including sexual, that has the potential for harm of the self or others [54, 55]. Within these general categories are many different behavioral syndromes that are well described and can be further explored in the literature [56].

Because agitation and aggression are common in AL, detection, prevention, and care are important [57]. The main precipitant of these behavioral expressions is cognitive stress or overload, suggesting that behaviors may be prevented by attending to these factors. Therefore, understanding the reasons why a resident with dementia may become agitated or aggressive is an important step toward person-centered care [58–60]. As summarized in Table 5.1, key reasons are grouped into three categories:

- noxious factors in the physical environment, such as lack of privacy; not feeling like home; a temperature that is too hot or cold; an uncomfortable chair; glare from bright lights on reflective surfaces; and noises such as alarms, staff shouting, and clanging dishes in the dining area;
- stressful aspects of the interpersonal environment, such as roommates; noisy public areas; and ungentle or uncomfortable personal care by staff; and
- internal (bodily) factors, such as constipation; thirst; hunger; a full bladder; wetness from incontinence; arthritis pain; spinal compression fractures; fatigue; depression; sleep deprivation; or boredom.

Detecting factors that trigger behavior expressions provides strategies to reduce them. For example, if a resident is bothered by loud sounds, moving them to a quieter space or providing headphones playing music that the resident enjoys may resolve

Table 5.1 Triggering factors (antecedents) for behavioral expressions in persons with Dementia

Type	Explanation	Examples
External, physical	The physical environment can be disorienting, unfamiliar, overcrowded, uncomfortable, or overstimulating	Lack of privacy; noise or glare; places that do not feel like home; showers that are too hot or too cold
External, interpersonal	Interactions with other residents, staff, or family can be frightening, demeaning, dismissive, or hurried	Daily care is being provided without explanation; being talked to an infantilizing manner; invalidating the perceptions of the persons with dementia
Internal	Biological needs and feelings can cause discomfort if they are unmet and difficult to communicate	Feelings of pain or hunger; illness; boredom; depression; delusions

distress—or even avoid it if done before the distress occurs. The *antecedent-behavior-consequence (ABC) assessment and management model* is useful to understand and address behavioral expressions; it posits that behavioral expressions are the consequence of antecedents that may be avoided, and evidence suggests that it is a useful model to employ in AL [61–64]. One multi-state AL study found that staff identified a potential cause for only a quarter of all behavioral expressions, but did so more often when they were able to successfully address the distress (i.e., 28% of the time in successfully managed cases compared to 20% of the time in unsuccessfully managed cases) [61]. Moreover, staff in dementia care units, and staff in smaller AL communities were more likely to identify antecedents, suggesting more familiarity promotes understanding of underlying unmet needs and can pave the way for a successful outcome for both residents and staff [61, 65].

Used systematically in AL, the ABC model can help determine which aspects of the environment and care might be modified. However, identifying antecedents can be challenging, so combining the ABC approach with the *habilitation approach* can be useful. The habilitation approach aims to maximize functional independence [62, 64], and similar to the ABC model, considers domains such as the environment and caregiving approaches, and proactively alters them to suit the needs of each individual without highlighting cognitive impairment [62]. This strategy can be helpful because it categorizes antecedents akin to a checklist, such as considering whether the antecedent was something in the physical environment, or a misperception of a caregiving encounter, or related to a conversation with another resident [62]. Thus, for assessment and management of behavioral expressions in persons with dementia, the combined ABC and habilitation approach may be helpful.

Medication and physical restraints, including psychoactive drugs, have historically been the dominant methods of controlling agitation and aggression in residents with dementia, but recent decades have seen increasing recognition of the need to prioritize non-pharmacologic, person-centered approaches [66]. Person-centered approaches aim to foster positive relationship-building and involve observations from staff, such as *emotion-oriented care* where staff receive training to employ empathy to understand the resident's perspective and gain knowledge of verbal and non-verbal communication [67]. Unfortunately, in the multi-state study noted above, the most common management strategy was the use of medications [61].

Overall, there is insufficient evidence as to whether pharmacologic approaches are at times more effective than behavioral ones at reducing aggression and agitation [66, 67], but even with lack of clear evidence, it is important to recognize that medications such as antipsychotics convey risks including strokes and movement disorders [66]. At the same time, there is an evidence base (albeit limited) that non-pharmacologic, person-centered approaches such as aromatherapy, music therapy, and structured care routines for bathing and mouth care can benefit overall well-being and reduce behavioral expressions, but the approaches must be tailored to each individual as not every person with dementia enjoys the same things or responds in the same manner [63].

Serious Mental Illness and Dementia in Assisted Living

In addition to being a primary care setting for persons with dementia, AL has a long history of housing persons with serious mental illness. The relationship between these populations is complex because behavioral expressions, such as verbal or physical aggression, or resistance to caregiving, are a feature of both. One study, for example, reported that 69% of AL residents with psychosis and 49% with dementia exhibited one or more behavioral expressions, including physical aggression in 30% of persons with psychosis and 19% of those with dementia [57].

Historically, persons with serious mental illness constituted a large proportion of AL residents because residential care facilities, which were the predecessors from which AL evolved, filled a gap created in the late 1960s and early 1970s by large-scale closure of psychiatric hospitals [68]. As of the mid-1980s, many residential care homes served exclusively persons with mental illness, and among those that did not specialize, 29% of their population had a history of a psychiatric hospitalization [69]. This concentration of serious mental illness in AL continued into the early 1990s, with a large national survey demonstrating that persons with chronic psychiatric conditions comprised 44% of residents, whereas persons with moderate to severe cognitive impairment comprised 40% [70]. In the late 1990s and early twenty-first century, however, as the nation's elderly population grew and nursing home construction was curtailed, AL boomed as an alternative setting for older adults with frailty and/or dementia. Thus, more recent data indicate that serious mental illness constitutes approximately 10% of the population and is much less prevalent than dementia [71].

The relationship between the serious mental illness legacy of AL and dementia care practices has not been studied, but it is possible that some traditions related to care of persons with chronic psychoses—such as antipsychotic use and referral to mental health centers—were extended to the care of behavioral expressions in persons with dementia [72]. If and when this occurs, it may relate to confusion about the two disorders. As a case in point, in the late 1990s during recruitment for a research study, our own team encountered two AL communities that claimed to be "dementia only" but exclusively housed persons with serious mental illness [73].

Today, the opposite is more likely the case, in that providers are often more well-informed about dementia than they are about serious mental illness, because persons with dementia are markedly more prevalent. A particularly complicating situation occurs when dementia and serious mental illness coexist. Thus, it is not surprising that coexistence of dementia and a chronic psychosis (schizophrenia or type 1 bipolar disorder) is associated with increased transfer from AL to nursing homes [74].

Specialized Units for People with Dementia

A contentious issue about dementia care in AL and other long-term care settings is the effectiveness of segregating residents with dementia from residents without dementia. This segregation can be achieved by housing residents with dementia in memory care units (also referred to as special care units; SCUs) or by employing environmental restraints (e.g., locked doors) that physically limit residents' movement and interaction with others [75]. At a community level, segregating residents with dementia in a setting that is entirely dedicated to memory care, or in a SCU within a larger community is not uncommon in the United States—20% of AL communities and 13% of nursing homes had this design in 2022; in AL, 11% of communities provided only memory care [20]. What constitutes memory care is not consistent across states, however, and many now specify what constitutes memory care in their AL legislation; common features include environmental design (e.g., 25 states have policies regarding egress), specialized staff training (e.g., 10 states require a designated administrator), and consumer disclosure (e.g., 33 states require disclosure of dementia-specific services) [76–80]. Notably, there has been an increase in states developing dementia care policies in memory care since 2007, including an increase in states requiring initial training of direct care workers and administrators, and cognitive screening of residents at the time of admission [81].

Research has produced limited evidence about the effectiveness of dementia SCUs. One recent review found no clear evidence that dementia SCUs improve outcomes of residents (e.g., social isolation), staff (e.g., burnout), families (e.g., satisfaction), or the long-term care community as a whole, but identified promising features needing additional study such as small-scale settings, specially trained staff, and multidisciplinary care approaches [82]. Another review found no strong evidence of any benefits of dementia SCUs, and concluded that improving care practice throughout the industry is likely more beneficial than segregation or specialization [79]. A third review found lower rates of new or worsening morbidity and hospitalizations in nursing home SCUs compared to non-SCUs, but reported greater functional decline in AL SCUs [26]. International studies also suggest that dementia SCUs do not significantly differ from traditional long-term care settings in terms of resident quality of life [83], nutritional status [84], type of care provided [85], and processes such as case conferences and mealtime practices [86, 87].

However, other studies suggest that dementia SCUs do offer benefits, such as more social engagement and less use of physical restraints, feeding tubes, pressure ulcers, and hospitalizations [76, 77, 88, 89]. Additionally, residents without dementia may prefer residing in communities that have segregated SCUs, especially if they remove residents with behavioral expressions such as wandering into others' rooms or making repetitive vocalizations [90]. Some studies also report lower rates of antipsychotic use in SCUs [77], but others report higher rates of prescribing [91, 92]. Most SCU research has been conducted in nursing homes, however, and lacks a focus on dementia SCUs in AL communities, which differ from nursing homes in important ways such as policies related to increased nursing staff and physician approval for admission to SCUs in AL [93–95]. That said, what research exists provides little evidence of a difference in outcome effectiveness for AL residents with dementia in SCUs versus non-specialized communities [93].

Related to the reason for varying findings, research about dementia SCUs has employed different methodologies. No precise definition of a dementia SCU exists, and models of care vary significantly, meaning that conclusions drawn from one study may not be widely generalizable [78, 82, 92]. Further, a randomized trial of special care is not feasible, and existing research at best attempts to statistically control for the fact that residents in dementia SCUs differ from residents with and without dementia in non-specialized settings (e.g., related to prognosis, behavioral expressions, physical function, and time since admission) [78, 79, 82, 91].

In addition to the controversy regarding SCU efficacy, the practice raises ethical concerns about autonomy, stigma, and cost. People with dementia value supports that promote independence, access to the outside world, options for family to visit and stay overnight, and freedom from walls and barriers—many of which are not typical of many SCUs [96, 97]. Additionally, the segregation of people with dementia from others may violate their human rights, specifically, the rights to non-discrimination, liberty and security, equality, accessibility, independent living, and community inclusion, all of which are delineated under the United Nations Convention on the Rights of Persons with Disabilities [75, 98]. Some research also suggests that SCU development is motivated by economic factors, such as attracting more private pay residents and promoting higher occupancy rates, resulting in a more costly option that may not be justified if SCUs do not provide better care [82, 91, 94].

Risk Management and Shared/Negotiated Risk Agreements in Assisted Living

Another contentious issue for dementia care in AL is the concept of risk, which is complicated by concerns about autonomous decision-making for people with dementia. Risk is conceptualized differently by individuals with dementia, those who provide their care, and health care professionals, in part based on their own experiences, life history, philosophy of life, and perspective on dementia [99–101]. Risk areas commonly discussed about persons with dementia include going outdoors alone (which may result in falls or becoming lost), driving (which may cause a vehicular accident), hobbies and occupations (such as gardening with inedible plants), and using potentially hazardous items (including candles, stoves, and sharp tools) [101].

Often, particularly among family and care providers, risk is viewed through an emotional lens and desire to protect the person with dementia, rather than as the probability of an outcome [99, 101]. This safety lens leads to a general desire to completely eliminate risk, an attitude that is especially prevalent in health care [102], rather than considering potential benefits, such as well-being associated with increased independence, control, and a sense of "normality" [100, 103–105]. Not surprisingly then, conflict can arise in AL between controlling risk and promoting autonomy and quality of life [86, 106], with staff reporting frustration at being asked to promote resident autonomy when they are concerned about the safety of residents whom they feel obligated to protect [107].

These issues are complicated by widespread assumptions about the decision-making abilities of people with dementia. Caregivers and family members often assume that a diagnosis of dementia, regardless of stage or progression, confers a loss of capacity for decision-making about one's health and other aspects of life [100, 108]. Such a perspective does not recognize that decision-making abilities and the values underlying them often remain until memory loss and other features of dementia are quite advanced [100], with a case in point being the right of a person with dementia who has smoked cigarettes for much of their life to continue doing so regardless of the health implications [109].

Best practice for risk assessment and management emphasizes seeking to involve individuals with dementia in decision-making and reaching a shared understanding of risk [101, 104]. If a person has the capacity to understand the issues, they should be allowed to make an informed choice about the risks and benefits of their behaviors [101]. The risk must be negotiated on an individual basis, as dementia does not affect everyone the same way, and constructions of risk vary depending on personal, cultural, and professional experiences [100, 104]. Further, risk assessment and management must be re-evaluated on a continuing basis, because they change over time [103, 104]. Overall, it is important to advocate for the active involvement of individuals with dementia in decision-making, especially because they are more likely to be overridden or excluded from decision-making about risks and medical care [110, 111].

One risk management strategy in AL is shared risk agreements, also known as negotiated risk agreements (NRA), which describe in writing the resident and family's understanding of the risks associated with the resident choices, typically those that conflict with medical or community guidelines. An NRA honors a resident's decision-making while managing its risks, presumably reducing liability, and producing a document that can be reviewed with the resident if they do not remember the conversation [112–114]. Common behaviors that prompt an NRA are drinking alcohol, smoking, refusing medications or bathing, and consuming foods high in sugar despite a diagnosis of diabetes [114].

NRAs are not without controversy, and no consensus exists about which behaviors and choices justify an NRA [107]. Opponents argue that NRAs are a way for AL communities to waive liability for negligence [115, 116]; proponents counter that NRAs do not prevent lawsuits or preclude safeguards against negligence [113]. Opponents highlight that residents already have the right to autonomy and should not have to negotiate away their rights or sign a document for their choices to be respected [113, 116]; proponents note that resident autonomy is often restricted in AL, especially due to liability concerns [107, 113]. Use of NRAs also raises concern about capacity, as it is unclear at what degree of cognitive impairment a resident loses the capacity to agree to an NRA [112, 117]. Finally, the terminology around NRAs is vague, inconsistently applied, and may be misused to justify substandard care [116]. Thus, risk and its management remains a challenging topic: there is a lack of a consistent legal framework for NRAs, and most states do not provide guidelines about them [107, 114, 117].

Partners Moving into Assisted Living When One Has Dementia

The majority of older adults wish to remain at home as they age, but physical and cognitive changes can make living at home difficult, especially for individuals without a partner [118]. Even for those with a partner, supportive AL care may become necessary when one has dementia [119], at which time the question becomes whether to move into AL together. If so, the intent may be complicated by factors such as availability of double rooms [120], admission criteria [1], differing care needs, and cost [118].

The reasons a couple may choose to remain together are numerous. Older adults, including people with dementia, value nonsexual intimacy and often report strong emotional and physical satisfaction with partner relationships [121, 122]. In these cases, couples may want to move to AL together so they can continue their closeness while one receives supportive care [119]. Also, adult children are often supportive of parents' decision to move together because it eases some of their concerns [123], and AL communities appreciate couples' desire to remain together, and many try to accommodate their request [119, 124].

The literature describes generally positive results when couples move to AL together [125], but there is considerable variation depending on individual factors such as sociability, support needed, and the quality of the couple's relationship [122, 123]. Smaller rooms, for example, can lead to friction more often than had been experienced in a larger home; however, the public spaces in AL may in part compensate for the smaller private space [123]. One main concern of couples living together is a lack of privacy from staff and other residents; measures to address this concern include locking doors and posting signs requesting knock before entry [123, 125]. Other challenges to joint residence are that most AL communities are designed for individuals rather than couples [123]; the cost of AL; and that many wait until a crisis occurs to consider moving to AL, sometimes leading to unwanted separation because immediately available options are limited [125]. Overall, although involuntary separation can cause grief, guilt, and failure—which is complicated due to changes in the behavior and communication of the person with dementia [126]—partners do tend to adjust to the separation [120].

Intimacy and Sexual Expression in Assisted Living Residents with Dementia

Sexuality, including the desire for touch and intimacy, is a normal human need, but when it involves AL residents with dementia the issue may be controversial. Even when AL is person-centered, sexual needs are often ignored and sometimes discouraged [12, 127, 128]. Sexual relations inherently raise legal issues of competence and consent and may also involve health issues such as risk of sexually transmitted diseases and injury.

Sexual expressions in AL range from intimate, nonsexual displays of affection such as holding hands or hugging another person to self-stimulation, unwanted verbal or physical advances on staff or other residents, and intimate sexual encounters [129]. Older adults, including AL residents with dementia, remain sexual beings, but most people with dementia and their partners value nonsexual intimacy more than sexual intimacy [127, 130, 131], with the prevalence and type of sexual expression depending on the individual [127, 129, 131, 132]. Among older adults with dementia, 46%–59% of men and 18%–51% of women are sexually active, with higher numbers related to those in a partnered relationship [133]. Self-stimulation occurs in roughly one quarter of men and 10% of women with dementia [133], but nonsexual intimate expressions occur in 70% [121, 134], and so should be recognized and supported [133, 134]. In fact, people with dementia actually rate nonsexual behaviors such as hugging and cuddling more favorably than intercourse [126]. Resident intimacy without intercourse is more accepted by AL staff than is intercourse, and as a result, those types of relationships exist more freely [135].

A number of concerns may arise about consent and possible exploitation of a resident with cognitive impairment, especially when a resident is unable to communicate abuse [136]. While staff may occasionally be the recipients of sexual overtures from residents with dementia, on rare occasions staff may initiate sexual intimacy themselves [135]. Another physical safety concern is the practice of safe sex between residents with dementia, including sexually transmitted infections [136, 137]. To maximize safety, AL staff and residents' families are advised to be aware of the sexual needs of people with dementia so they can support safe-sex practices in consenting couples [136, 137].

The most important issue surrounding sexual expression for people with dementia in AL is the concept of capacity and consent, specifically whether the resident is able to give or withhold consent to a relationship and physical intimacy, which may depend on the stage of disease [128, 136, 138]. There is also variation by state as to what determines capacity; some states require that a person only understands physical intercourse and participate voluntarily, while other states require understanding of sexually transmitted diseases, or even an understanding of moral and social consequences [136]. AL staff are frequently in a position of having to assess capacity to consent, and when that is necessary, participant understanding, reasoning, and engaging voluntarily are generally agreed upon criteria [128, 136, 139].

Family attitudes also weigh in when sexual expression is involved, especially when a new relationship develops between two residents and one or both has cognitive impairment [127, 128, 140, 141]. Some families may appreciate that their relative has found companionship in the AL community, but others may have concerns that the activity is not consistent with the resident's previous behavior; that true consent is not possible; that physical harm could occur; or that exploitation may be involved. Such concerns can influence decision-making in ways that override a resident's autonomy, especially if a concerned family member has power of attorney or is financially responsible for the AL stay [127, 128, 136, 137]. When relationships continue despite family objection, and especially if they become sexual, families may threaten the AL community with legal action or transfer to another community [127, 140, 141].

In light of these challenges, AL communities are recommended to have policies in place for sexual activity; however, not all do, and even fewer have specific policies for residents with dementia [128, 134, 136]. In practice, AL communities generally prefer informal approaches to intimacy and sexual expression and because of legal concerns, incline toward conservative views toward residents' sexual expressions [128, 136, 140, 142]. Unfortunately, informal approaches open the door for conflict between families and staff and can lead to legal challenges [128].

Implications for "Assisted" and "Living"

As the primary provider of long-term residential care for persons with dementia who can no longer reside at home or with family, AL communities face unique challenges and opportunities. This chapter outlined some of those challenges, including understanding the cognitive status of each AL resident, identifying and addressing each person's unique care needs, fostering positive engagement, understanding and dealing with behavioral expressions, and addressing a variety of special situations such as coexisting serious mental illness, risk management, accommodating cognitively intact partners, and issues related to intimacy and sexuality. In serving this complex population, the summative question is "to what extent does AL promote 'assisted' and 'living' for person with dementia?".

Because persons with dementia require supportive care, a focus on "assisted" is central to dementia care. Each person with cognitive impairment has unique abilities and needs, such that assistive care requires the AL community to have a suitable number of well-trained staff, and supportive leadership, to individualize the assistance provided. Cognitive and physical assistance should include environmental components that orient and engage, and staff who use language and care approaches appropriate to each resident's' abilities and needs. Staffing is critical to providing that assistance, and the number and mix of staff must fit residents' needs. Given pervasive staffing challenges, AL communities must work efficiently within their resources to maximize their ability to assist all residents.

Optimizing "living" is even more complex, because the unresolved issues discussed in this chapter speak not just about "care" but about attending to the ethical and humane aspects of life in a residential community. Ideally, all residents should have optimal quality of life in an environment that addresses physical needs; provides safety, security, and social engagement; and fosters self-esteem according to individual wishes and preferences. However, AL is a group setting, and living in a community creates limitations on personal freedom. Further, AL residents have impairments that limit their ability to live as they would prefer, and staff have limitations in terms of time and resources. Therefore, optimizing "living" in AL requires more than an informed workforce and facilitative environment; it requires involvement and advocacy from a range of constituencies—family, community and industry leadership, advocacy groups, and enlightened regulation—each invested in the well-being of all AL residents, especially those with dementia who cannot effectively advocate for themselves.

Competing Interests The authors have no conflicts of interest to declare that are relevant to the content of this chapter.

References

1. Zimmerman S, Sloane PD, Reed D. Dementia prevalence and care in assisted living. Health Aff (Millwood). 2014 Apr;33(4):658–66. https://doi.org/10.1377/hlthaff.2013.1255.
2. Sachdev PS, Blacker D, Blazer DG, Ganguli M, Jeste DV, Paulsen JS, Petersen RC. Classifying neurocognitive disorders: the DSM-5 approach. Nat Rev Neurol. 2014 Nov;10(11):634–42. https://doi.org/10.1038/nrneurol.2014.181.
3. Pérez Palmer N, Trejo Ortega B, Joshi P. Cognitive impairment in older adults: epidemiology, diagnosis, and treatment. Psychiatr Clin North Am. 2022 Dec;45(4):639–61. https://doi.org/10.1016/j.psc.2022.07.010.
4. Erkkinen MG, Kim MO, Geschwind MD. Clinical neurology and epidemiology of the major neurodegenerative diseases. Cold Spring Harb Perspect Biol. 2018 Apr;10(4):1–44. https://doi.org/10.1101/cshperspect.a033118.
5. O'Brien JT, Thomas A. Vascular dementia. Lancet. 2015 Oct;386(10004):1698–706. https://doi.org/10.1016/S0140-6736(15)00463-8.
6. Chodosh J, Edelen MO, Buchanan JL, Yosef JA, Ouslander JG, Berlowitz DR, Streim JE, Saliba D. Nursing home assessment of cognitive impairment: development and testing of a brief instrument of mental status. J Am Geriatr Soc. 2008 Nov;56(11):2069–75. https://doi.org/10.1111/j.1532-5415.2008.01944.x.

7. Melekin A, Sengupta M, Caffrey C. Residential care community resident characteristics: United States, 2022. NCHS Data Brief. 2024 Aug;506:1–9. https://doi.org/10.15620/cdc/158327.
8. Caffrey C, Melekin A, Lu Z, Sengupta M. Variation in residential care community resident characteristics, by size of community: United States, 2020. NCHS Data Brief. 2022;454:1–8. https://doi.org/10.15620/cdc:121910.
9. Spillman BC, Liu K, McGillard C. Trends in residential long-term care: use of nursing homes and assisted living and characteristics of facilities and residents. U.S. Department of Health and Human Services. November 24, 2002. https://aspe.hhs.gov/sites/default/files/private/pdf/72746/rltct.pdf. Accessed July 4, 2025.
10. Hafiz R, Alajlani L, Ali A, Algarni GA, Aljurfi H, Alammar OA, Ashqan MY, Alkhashan A. The latest advances in the diagnosis and treatment of dementia. Cureus. 2023 Dec;15(12):1–9. https://doi.org/10.7759/cureus.50522.
11. Wilson KB. Historical evolution of assisted living in the United States, 1979 to the present. Gerontologist. 2007 Dec;47(suppl 1):8–22. https://doi.org/10.1093/geront/47.supplement_1.8.
12. Zimmerman S. Toward a common definition of assisted living. [Internet]. McKnights Senior Living; 2024 Sept 3 [cited 2025 Jul 03]. Available from: https://www.mcknightsseniorliving.com/home/columns/guest-columns/toward-a-common-definition-of-assisted-living/
13. Zimmerman S, Sloane PD, Williams CS, Dobbs D, Ellajosyula R, Braaten A, Rupnow MF, Kaufer DI. Residential care/assisted living staff may detect undiagnosed dementia using the minimum data set cognition scale. J Am Geriatr Soc. 2007 Sep;55(9):1349–55. https://doi.org/10.1111/j.1532-5415.2007.01289.x.
14. King M, Peckham A, Marani H, Roerig M, Yung S, McGrail K, Young Y, Shaw J, Marchildon G. Gaps in the system: supporting people living with dementia. J Aging Soc Policy. 2023 Jul;36(5):963–83. https://doi.org/10.1080/08959420.2023.2226341.
15. Fernando E, Fraser M, Hendriksen J, Kim CH, Muir-Hunter SW. Risk factors associated with falls in older adults with dementia: a systematic review. Physiother Can. 2017;69(2):161–70. https://doi.org/10.3138/ptc.2016-14.
16. Hyde J, Perez R, Forester B. Dementia and assisted living. Gerontologist. 2007;47(suppl 1):51–67. https://doi.org/10.1093/geront/47.
17. Ciofi JM, Kemp CL, Bender AA. Assisted living residents with dementia: being out in the world and negotiating connections. Gerontologist. 2021 Aug;62(2):200–11. https://doi.org/10.1093/geront/gnab113.
18. Day K, Cohen U. The role of culture in designing environments for people with dementia: a study of Russian Jewish immigrants. Environ Behav. 2000 May;32(3):361–99. https://doi.org/10.1177/00139160021972577.
19. Sloane PD, Zimmerman S, Gruber-Baldini AL, Hebel R, Magaziner J, Konrad TR. Health and functional outcomes and health care utilization of persons with dementia in residential care and assisted living facilities: comparison with nursing homes. Gerontologist. 2005 Oct;45(suppl 1):124–34. https://doi.org/10.1093/geront/45.suppl_1.124.
20. National Center for Health Statistics. Data from the national post-acute and long-term care study [Internet]. CDC; 2020 [cited 2025 Aug 04]. Available from: https://www.cdc.gov/nchs/npals/webtables/overview.htm
21. Manis DR, Rahim A, Poss JW, Bielska IA, Bronskill SE, Tarride JE, Abelson J, Costa AP. Do assisted living facilities that offer a dementia care program differ from those that do not? A population-level cross-sectional study in Ontario, Canada. BMC Geriatr. 2021 Aug;21:1–7. https://doi.org/10.1186/s12877-021-02400-w.
22. Beeber AS, Zimmerman S, Reed D, Mitchell CM, Sloane PD, Harris-Wallace B, Perez R, Schumacher JG. Licensed nurse staffing and health service availability in residential care and assisted living. J Am Geriatr Soc. 2014 May;62(5):805–11. https://doi.org/10.1111/jgs.12786.
23. Beeber AS, Zimmerman S, Mitchell CM, Reed D. Staffing and service availability in assisted living: the importance of nurse delegation policies. J Am Geriatr Soc. 2018 Nov;66(11):2158–66. https://doi.org/10.1111/jgs.15580.

24. Unroe KT, Bernard B, Stump TE, Tu W, Callahan CM. Variation in hospice services by location of care: nursing home versus assisted living facility versus home. J Am Geriatr Soc. 2017 Jul;65(7):1490–6. https://doi.org/10.1111/jgs.14826.
25. Unroe KT, Stump TE, Effler S, Tu W, Callahan CM. Quality of hospice care at home versus in an assisted living facility or nursing home. J Am Geriatr Soc. 2018 Apr;66(4):687–92. https://doi.org/10.1111/jgs.15260.
26. Zimmerman S, Anderson WL, Brode S, Jonas D, Lux L, Beeber AS, Watson LC, Viswanathan M, Lohr KN, Sloane PD. Systematic review: Effective characteristics of nursing homes and other residential long-term care settings for people with dementia. J Am Geriatr Soc. 2013 Aug;61(8):1399–409. https://doi.org/10.1111/jgs.12372.
27. National Academies of Sciences, Engineering, and Medicine. The national imperative to improve nursing home quality: honoring our commitment to residents, families, and staff. Washington, DC: The National Academies Press; 2022. https://doi.org/10.17226/26526.
28. Kaup ML, Calkins MP, Davey A, Wrublowsky R. The environmental audit screening evaluation: establishing reliability and validity of an evidence-based design tool. Innov Aging. 2023 Apr;7(5):1–12. https://doi.org/10.1093/geroni/igad039.
29. Namazi KH, Johnson BD. Environmental effects on incontinence problems in Alzheimer's disease patients. American Journal of Alzheimer's Care and Related Disorders & Research. 1991;6(6):16–21. https://doi.org/10.1177/153331759100600604.
30. Calkins MP. Evidence-based long term care design. NeuroRehabilitation. 2009;25(3):145–54. https://doi.org/10.3233/NRE-2009-0512.
31. Rocha V, Marques A, Pinto M, Sousa L, Figueiredo D. People with dementia in long-term care facilities: an exploratory study of their activities and participation. Disabil Rehabil. 2013 Aug;35(18):1501–8. https://doi.org/10.3109/09638288.2012.742677.
32. Zimmerman S, Allen J, Cohen LW, Pinkowitz J, Reed D, Coffey WO, Reed P, Lepore M, Sloane PD. A measure of person-centered practices in assisted living: the PC-PAL. J Am Med Dir Assoc. 2015 Feb;16(2):132–7. https://doi.org/10.1016/j.jamda.2014.07.016.
33. Kitwood T. Dementia reconsidered: the person comes first. London: Open University Press; 1997.
34. Zimmerman S, Cohen LW, Reed D, Gwyther LP, Washington T, Cagle JG, Sloane PD, Preisser JS. Families matter in long-term care: results of a group-randomized trial. Seniors Hous Care J. 2013;21(1):3–20.
35. Hall GR, Buckwalter KC. Progressively lowered stress threshold: a conceptual model for care of adults with Alzheimer's disease. Arch Psychiatr Nurs. 1987 Dec;1(6):399–406.
36. Mansbach WE, Mace RA, Clark KM, Firth IM. Meaningful activity for long-term care residents with dementia: a comparison of activities and raters. Gerontologist. 2017 Jun;57(3):461–8. https://doi.org/10.1093/geront/gnv694.
37. Han A, Radel J, McDowd JM, Sabata D. Perspectives of people with dementia about meaningful activities: a synthesis. Am J Alzheimers Dis Other Demen. 2016 Mar;31(2):115–23. https://doi.org/10.1177/1533317515598857.
38. Roland KP, Chappell NL. Meaningful activity for persons with dementia: family caregiver perspectives. Am J Alzheimers Dis Other Demen. 2015 Sep;30(6):559–68. https://doi.org/10.1177/1533317515576389.
39. Phinney A, Chaudhury H, O'Connor DL. Doing as much as I can do: the meaning of activity for people with dementia. Aging Ment Health. 2007 Jul;11(4):384–93. https://doi.org/10.1080/13607860601086470.
40. Reed P, Tilly J. Dementia care practice recommendations for nursing homes and assisted living, phase 1: dementia care fundamentals, food and fluid consumption, pain management, and social engagement. Alzheimers Care Today. 2008 Mar;9(1):33.
41. Kemp CL, Bender AA, Morgan JC, Burgess EO, Epps FR, Hill AM, Perkins MM. Understanding capacity and optimizing meaningful engagement among persons living with dementia. Dementia. 2023 May;22(4):854–74. https://doi.org/10.1177/14713012231162713.
42. Fazio S, Pace D, Flinner J, Kallmyer B. The fundamentals of person-centered care for individuals with dementia. Gerontologist. 2018 Jan;58(suppl 1):S10–9. https://doi.org/10.1093/geront/gnx122.

43. Holopainen A, Siltanen H, Pohjanvuori A, Mäkisalo-Ropponen M, Okkonen E. Factors associated with the quality of life of people with dementia and with quality of life-improving interventions: scoping review. Dementia. 2019 May;18(4):1507–37. https://doi.org/10.1177/1471301217716725.
44. Theurer K, Mortenson WB, Stone R, Suto M, Timonen V, Rozanova J. The need for a social revolution in residential care. J Aging Stud. 2015 Dec;35:201–10. https://doi.org/10.1016/j.jaging.2015.08.011.
45. Trahan MA, Kuo J, Carlson MC, Gitlin LN. A systematic review of strategies to foster activity engagement in persons with dementia. Health Educ Behav. 2014 Oct;41(suppl 1):70S-83S. https://doi.org/10.1177/1090198114531782.
46. Buettner LL, Fitzsimmons S. Activity calendars for older adults with dementia: what you see is not what you get. Am J Alzheimers Dis Other Demen. 2003 Jul;18(4):215–26. https://doi.org/10.1177/153331750301800405.
47. Kemp CL, Bender AA, Ciofi J, Morgan JC, Burgess EO, Duong S, Epps FR, Hill AM, Manley PR, Sease J, Perkins MM. Meaningful engagement among assisted living residents with dementia: successful approaches. J Appl Gerontol. 2021 Dec;40(12):1751–7. https://doi.org/10.1177/0733464821996866.
48. Smith N, Towers AM, Palmer S, Beecham J, Welch E. Being occupied: supporting 'meaningful activity' in care homes for older people in England. Ageing Soc. 2018 Nov;38(11):2218–40. https://doi.org/10.1017/S0144686X17000678.
49. Kontos P, Grigorovich A, Kosurko A, Bar RJ, Herron RV, Menec VH, Skinner MW. Dancing with dementia: exploring the embodied dimensions of creativity and social engagement. Gerontologist. 2021 Aug;61(5):714–23. https://doi.org/10.1093/geront/gnaa129.
50. Zimmerman S, Stone R, Carder P, Thomas K. Does assisted living provide assistance and promote living? Health Aff. 2024 May;43(5):674–81. https://doi.org/10.1377/hlthaff.2023.00972.
51. Neal I, du Toit SH, Lovarini M. The use of technology to promote meaningful engagement for adults with dementia in residential aged care: a scoping review. Int Psychogeriatr. 2020 Aug;32(8):913–35. https://doi.org/10.1017/S1041610219001388.
52. Macaulay S. The Broken Lens of BPSD: Why We Need to Rethink the Way We Label the Behavior of People Who Live with Alzheimer Disease. J Am Med Dir Assoc. 2018 Feb;19(2):177–80.
53. Gilmore MC, Stebbins L, Arguelles-Borge S, Trinidad B, Golden CJ. Development and treatment of aggression in individuals with dementia. Aggress Violent Behav. 2020 Sep;54:1–12. https://doi.org/10.1016/j.avb.2020.101415.
54. Wong B, Wu P, Ismail Z, Watt J, Goodarzi Z. Detecting agitation and aggression in persons living with dementia: a systematic review of diagnostic accuracy. BMC Geriat. 2024 Jun;24(1):1–18. https://doi.org/10.1186/s12877-024-05143-6.
55. Gimm G, Chowdhury S, Castle N. Resident aggression and abuse in assisted living. J Appl Gerontol. 2018 Aug;37(8):947–64. https://doi.org/10.1177/0733464816661947.
56. Cohen-Mansfield J, Marx MS, Rosenthal AS. A description of agitation in a nursing home. J Gerontol. 1989;44(3):M77–84. https://doi.org/10.1093/geronj/44.3.m77.
57. Gruber-Baldini AL, Boustani M, Sloane PD, Zimmerman S. Behavioral symptoms in residential care/assisted living facilities: prevalence, risk factors, and medication management. J Am Geriatr Soc. 2004 Oct;52(10):1610–7. https://doi.org/10.1111/j.1532-5415.2004.52451.x.
58. Grigorovich A, Kontos P, Kontos AP. The "violent resident": a critical exploration of the ethics of resident-to-resident aggression. J Bioeth Inq. 2019 Feb;16:173–83. https://doi.org/10.1007/s11673-019-09898-1.
59. Stutte K, Hahn S, Fierz K, Zuniga F. Factors associated with aggressive behavior between residents and staff in nursing homes. Geriatr Nurs. 2017 Sep;38(5):398–405. https://doi.org/10.1016/j.gerinurse.2017.02.001.
60. Volicer L. Behavioral problems and dementia. Clin Geriatr Med. 2018 Nov;34(4):637–51. https://doi.org/10.1016/j.cger.2018.06.009.

61. Dobbs D, Zimmerman S, Carder P, Beeber AS, Palmertree SJ. Staff reports of behavioral expressions of persons with dementia in 250 assisted living communities. Gerontologist. 2022 Feb;62(2):169–80. https://doi.org/10.1093/geront/gnab059.
62. Volicer L, Hurley AC. Review article: management of behavioral symptoms in progressive degenerative dementias. J Gerontol A Biol Sci Med Sci. 2003 Sep;58(9):M837–45. https://doi.org/10.1093/gerona/58.9.m837.
63. Warren A. BPSD reconsidered: diagnostic considerations to preserve personhood in persons with dementia. Front Dement. 2023 Nov;2:1–8. https://doi.org/10.3389/frdem.2023.1272400.
64. Kitwood T. Person and process in dementia. Int J Geriatr Psychiatry. 1993 Jul;8(7):541–5. https://doi.org/10.1002/gps.930080702.
65. McKenzie G, Teri L, Pike K, LaFazia D, van Leynseele J. Reactions of assisted living staff to behavioral and psychological symptoms of dementia. Geriatr Nurs. 2012 Mar;33(2):96–104. https://doi.org/10.1016/j.gerinurse.2011.12.004.
66. Watt JA, Porter J, Tavilsup P, Chowdhury M, Hatch S, Ismail Z, Kumar S, Kirkham J, Goodarzi Z, Seitz D. Guideline recommendations on behavioral and psychological symptoms of dementia: a systematic review. J Am Med Dir Assoc. 2024 May;25(5):837–46. https://doi.org/10.1016/j.jamda.2024.03.007.
67. Jutkowitz E, Brasure M, Fuchs E, Shippee T, Kane RA, Fink HA, Butler M, Sylvanus T, Kane RL. Care-delivery interventions to manage agitation and aggression in dementia nursing home and assisted living residents: a systematic review and meta-analysis. J Am Geriatr Soc. 2016 Mar;64(3):477–88. https://doi.org/10.1111/jgs.13936.
68. Morgan LA, Perez R, Frankowski AC, Nemec M, Bennett CR. Mental illness in assisted living: challenges for quality of life and care. J Hous Elderly. 2016;30(2):185–98. https://doi.org/10.1080/02763893.2016.1162255.
69. Mor V, Sherwood S, Gutkin C. A national study of residential care for the aged. Gerontologist. 1986 Aug;26(4):405–17. https://doi.org/10.1093/geront/26.4.405.
70. Hawes C, Wildfire J, Mor V, Wilcox V, Spore D, Iannacchione V, Lux L, Green R, Greene A, Phillips C. A description of board and care facilities, operators, and residents. Report to the Assistant Secretary for Planning and Evaluation. Research Triangle Park, NC. US Department of Health and Human Services, Research Triangle Institute, and Brown University; December 1995.
71. Hua CL, Cornell PY, Zimmerman S, Winfree J, Thomas KS. Trends in serious mental illness in US assisted living compared to nursing homes and the community: 2007–2017. Am J Geriatr Psychiatry. 2021 May;29(5):434–44. https://doi.org/10.1016/j.jagp.2020.09.011.
72. Sloane P, Mutran E, Sharp J, Hargett F, Hatch J. Domiciliary care in North Carolina: effect of home size, urban/rural status, and racial composition. Gerontologist. 1995 Oct;35(1):1–464. https://doi.org/10.1093/geront/35.Special_Issue_I.1.
73. Davis KJ, Sloane PD, Mitchell CM, Preisser J, Grant L, Hawes MC, Lindeman D, Montgomery R, Phillips C, Long KM, Koch G. Specialized dementia programs in residential care settings. Gerontologist. 2000 Feb;40(1):32–42. https://doi.org/10.1093/geront/40.1.32.
74. Temkin-Greener H, Guo W, McGarry B, Cai S. Serious mental illness in assisted living communities: association with nursing home placement. J Am Med Dir Assoc. 2024 May;25(5):917–22. https://doi.org/10.1016/j.jamda.2024.02.015.
75. Steele L, Swaffer K, Phillipson L, Fleming R. Questioning segregation of people living with dementia in Australia: an international human rights approach to care homes. Laws. 2019 Sep;8(3):18. https://doi.org/10.3390/laws8030018.
76. Adlbrecht L, Nemeth T, Frommlet F, Bartholomeyczik S, Mayer H. Engagement in purposeful activities and social interactions amongst persons with dementia in special care units compared to traditional nursing homes: an observational study. Scand J Caring Sci. 2022 Sep;36(3):650–62. https://doi.org/10.1111/scs.13017.
77. Joyce NR, McGuire TG, Bartels SJ, Mitchell SL, Grabowski DC. The impact of dementia special care units on quality of care: an instrumental variables analysis. Health Serv Res. 2018;53(5):3657–79. https://doi.org/10.1111/1475-6773.12867.

78. Palm R, Fahsold A, Roes M, Holle B. Context, mechanisms and outcomes of dementia special care units: an initial programme theory based on realist methodology. PLoS ONE. 2021 Nov;16(11):1–22. https://doi.org/10.1371/journal.pone.0259496.
79. Lai CK, Yeung JH, Mok V, Chi I. Special care units for dementia individuals with behavioural problems. Cochrane Database Syst Rev. 2009;(4):CD006470. https://doi.org/10.1002/14651858.CD006470.pub2.
80. Carder PC. State regulatory approaches for dementia care in residential care and assisted living. Gerontologist. 2017 Aug;57(4):776–86. https://doi.org/10.1093/geront/gnw197.
81. Smith L, Carder P, Bucy T, Winfree J, Brazier JF, Kaskie B, Thomas KS. Connecting policy to licensed assisted living communities, introducing health services regulatory analysis. Health Serv Res. 2021 Jun;56(3):540–9. https://doi.org/10.1111/1475-6773.13616.
82. Orth J, Flowers D, Betz G, Cagle JG. A systematic review of specialty dementia care units in long-term care settings. Int J Geriatr Psychiatry. 2023 Apr;38(4):1–28. https://doi.org/10.1002/gps.5907.
83. Mjørud M, Kirkevold M, Røsvik J, Selbæk G, Engedal K. Variables associated to quality of life among nursing home patients with dementia. Aging Ment Health. 2014;18(8):1013–21. https://doi.org/10.1080/13607863.2014.903468.
84. Aukner C, Eide HD, Iversen PO. Nutritional status among older residents with dementia in open versus special care units in municipal nursing homes: an observational study. BMC Geriatr. 2013 Mar;13:26. https://doi.org/10.1186/1471-2318-13-26.
85. Crespo M, Hornillos C, Gómez MM. Dementia special care units: a comparison with standard units regarding residents' profile and care features. Int Psychogeriatr. 2013 Dec;25(12):2023–31. https://doi.org/10.1017/S1041610213001439.
86. Palm R, Trutschel D, Simon M, Bartholomeyczik S, Holle B. Differences in case conferences in dementia specific vs traditional care units in German nursing homes: results from a cross-sectional study. J Am Med Dir Assoc. 2016 Jan;17(1):91.e9-13. https://doi.org/10.1016/j.jamda.2015.08.018.
87. Milte R, Bradley C, Miller M, Farrer O, Crotty M. How widely are supportive and flexible food service systems and mealtime interventions used for people in residential care facilities? A comparison of dementia-specific and nonspecific facilities. Healthcare (Basel). 2018 Dec;6(4):140. https://doi.org/10.3390/healthcare6040140.
88. Beerens HC, Zwakhalen SM, Verbeek H, Tan FE, Jolani S, Downs M, de Boer B, Ruwaard D, Hamers JP. The relation between mood, activity, and interaction in long-term dementia care. Aging Ment Health. 2018 Jan;22(1):26–32. https://doi.org/10.1080/13607863.2016.1227766.
89. Adlbrecht L, Bartholomeyczik S, Hildebrandt C, Mayer H. Social interactions of persons with dementia living in special care units in long-term care: a mixed-methods systematic review. Dementia. 2021 Apr;20(3):967–84. https://doi.org/10.1177/1471301220919937.
90. Calkins MP. From research to application: supportive and therapeutic environments for people living with dementia. Gerontologist. 2018 Jan;58(suppl 1):S114–28. https://doi.org/10.1093/geront/gnx146.
91. Gruneir A, Lapane KL, Miller SC, Mor V. Is dementia special care really special? A new look at an old question. J Am Geriatr Soc. 2008;56(2):199–205. https://doi.org/10.1111/j.1532-5415.2007.01559.x.
92. Cadigan RO, Grabowski DC, Givens JL, Mitchell SL. The quality of advanced dementia care in the nursing home: the role of special care units. Med Care. 2012 Oct;50(10):856–62. https://doi.org/10.1097/MLR.0b013e31825dd713.
93. Samus QM, Mayer L, Baker A, McNabney M, Brandt J, Onyike CU, Rabins PV, Lyketsos CG, Rosenblatt A. Characteristics and outcomes for assisted living residents with dementia: comparing dementia-specific care units with non-dementia-specific care units. J Am Geriatr Soc. 2008 Jul;56(7):1361–3. https://doi.org/10.1111/j.1532-5415.2008.01722.x.
94. Zimmerman S, Gruber-Baldini AL, Sloane PD, Eckert JK, Hebel JR, Morgan LA, Stearns SC, Wildfire J, Magaziner J, Chen C, Konrad TR. Assisted living and nursing homes: apples and oranges? Gerontologist. 2003 Apr;43(suppl 2):107–17. https://doi.org/10.1093/geront/43.suppl_2.107.

95. Elliot AE, Bowblis JR, Nelson I, Menne H. What happens behind closed doors? Investigating care practices in nursing home and assisted living memory care units. Health Aff Sch. 2025 Feb;3(2):1–6. https://doi.org/10.1093/haschl/qxaf026.
96. Swaffer K. What people with dementia want from residential care homes [Internet]. 2016 [cited 2024 Jul 9]. Available from: https://www.agedcarecrisis.com/opinion/articles/370-what-people-with-dementia-want-from-residential-care-homes
97. Steele L, Carr R, Swaffer K, Phillipson L, Fleming R. Human rights and the confinement of people living with dementia in care homes. Health Hum Rights. 2020 Jun;22(1):7–19.
98. Swaffer K. Human rights, disability and dementia. Aust J Dement Care. 2018 Feb;7(1):25–8.
99. Hoe J, Profyri E, Kemp C, Manela M, Webster L, Anthony J, Costafreda S, Arrojo F, Souris H, Livingston G. Risk assessment for people living with dementia: a systematic review. Int Psychogeriatr. 2024 Apr;36(4):263–88. https://doi.org/10.1017/S1041610223004398.
100. Dickins M, Goeman D, O'Keefe F, Iliffe S, Pond D. Understanding the conceptualisation of risk in the context of community dementia care. Soc Sci Med. 2018 Jul;208:72–9. https://doi.org/10.1016/j.socscimed.2018.05.018.
101. Stevenson M, Savage B, Taylor BJ. Perception and communication of risk in decision making by persons with dementia. Dementia. 2019 Apr;18(3):1108–27. https://doi.org/10.1177/1471301217704119.
102. Robinson L, Hutchings D, Corner L, Finch T, Hughes J, Brittain K, Bond J. Balancing rights and risks: conflicting perspectives in the management of wandering in dementia. Health Risk Soc. 2007 Dec;9(4):389–406. https://doi.org/10.1080/13698570701612774.
103. Calkins M, Brush J. Honoring individual choice in long-term residential communities when it involves risk: a person-centered approach. J Gerontol Nurs. 2016 Aug;42(8):12–7. https://doi.org/10.3928/00989134-20160531-01.
104. Manthorpe J, Moriarty J. 'Nothing ventured, nothing gained': risk guidance for people with dementia [Internet]. 2010 [cited 2024 Jul 15] Available from https://www.gov.uk/government/publications/nothing-ventured-nothing-gained-risk-guidance-for-people-with-dementia
105. Mitchell W, Glendinning C. A review of the research evidence surrounding risk perceptions, risk management strategies and their consequences in adult social care for different groups of service users. University of York, York: Social Policy Research Unit, University of York; 2007.
106. Clarke CL, Gibb CE, Keady J, Luce A, Wilkinson H, Williams L, Cook A. Risk management dilemmas in dementia care: an organizational survey in three UK countries. Int J Older People Nurs. 2009;4(2):89–96. https://doi.org/10.1111/j.1748-3743.2008.00149.x.
107. Jenkens R, O'Keefe J, Carder P, Brown Wilson K. A study of negotiated risk agreements in assisted living: final report [Internet] ASPE; 2006 [cited 2024 Jul 14]. Available from: https://aspe.hhs.gov/reports/study-negotiated-risk-agreements-assisted-living-final-report-1
108. Carr S. Enabling risk and ensuring safety: self-directed support and personal budgets. J of Adult Prot. 2010;13(3):122–36. https://doi.org/10.1108/14668201111160723.
109. Clarke C, Keady J, Wilkinson H, Gibb C, Luce A, Cook A, Williams L. Dementia and risk: contested territories of everyday life. J Nurs Healthc Chronic Illn. 2010 May;2(2):102–12. https://doi.org/10.1111/j.1752-9824.2010.01040.x.
110. Miller LM, Whitlatch CJ, Lyons KS. Shared decision-making in dementia: a review of patient and family carer involvement. Dementia. 2016 Sep;15(5):1141–57. https://doi.org/10.1177/1471301214555542.
111. Fetherstonhaugh D, Tarzia L, Nay R. Being central to decision making means I am still here!: the essence of decision making for people with dementia. J Aging Stud. 2013 Apr;27(2):143–50. https://doi.org/10.1016/j.jaging.2012.12.007.
112. Grubman JF. Methods for managing risk and promoting resident-centered care in nursing homes. Columbia J Law Soc Probl. 2015;49(2):217–49.
113. Mitty E, Flores S. Aging in place and negotiated risk agreements. Geriatr Nurs. 2008;29(2):94–101. https://doi.org/10.1016/j.gerinurse.2008.01.001.

114. Negotiated risk agreements: when and how should they be used? [Internet]. CNA; 2019 [cited 2025 Jul 03]. Available from: https://www.cna.com/web/wcm/connect/eac223d5-5b6a-424b-8e5c-5538c9350a1c/CNA-Carefully-Speaking-Negotiated-Risk-Agreements.pdf?MOD=AJPERES&CACHEID=eac223d5-5b6a-424b-8e5c-5538c9350a1c
115. Carlson EM. Negotiating for resident-centered care. Marquette Elder's Advisor. 2012;10(1):21–54.
116. Carlson EM. Protecting rights or waiving them? Why "negotiated risk" should be removed from assisted living law. J Health Care Law Policy. 2007 Jan 1;10(2):287.
117. Carder P, O'Keeffe J, O'Keeffe C. Compendium of residential care and assisted living regulations and policy: 2015 edition. ASPE; 2015 Jun 14 [cited 2025 Jul 03]. Available from: https://aspe.hhs.gov/reports/compendium-residential-care-assisted-living-regulations-policy-2015-edition-0
118. Thomeer MB, Mudrazija S, Angel JL. Relationship status and long-term care facility use in later life. J Gerontol B Psychol Sci Soc Sci. 2015 Nov;71(4):711–23. https://doi.org/10.1093/geronb/gbv106.
119. Howley EK. Assisted living for couples: what you need to know [Internet]. U.S. News; 2024 Aug 26 [cited 2025 Jun 12]. Available from: https://health.usnews.com/best-senior-living/assisted-living/articles/assisted-living-for-couples
120. Glasier W, Arbeau K, Launeanu M, Kwee J. The social process of involuntary separation and the search for connection. Health Psychol Open. 2024 Apr;11:1–16. https://doi.org/10.1177/20551029231224368.
121. Davies HD, Sridhar SB, Newkirk LA, Beaudreau SA, O'Hara R. Gender differences in sexual behaviors of AD patients and their relationship to spousal caregiver well-being. Aging Ment Health. 2011 Oct;16(1):89–101. https://doi.org/10.1080/13607863.2011.609532.
122. Kemp CL, Ball MM, Perkins MM. Couples' social careers in assisted living: reconciling individual and shared situations. Gerontologist. 2016 Oct;56(5):841–54. https://doi.org/10.1093/geront/gnv025.
123. Kemp CL. Married couples in assisted living: adult children's experiences providing support. J Fam Issues. 2012 May;33(5):639–61. https://doi.org/10.1177/0192513X11416447.
124. Marcus J. Couples with Different Health Needs Can Now Live Together in Some Long-Term Care Facilities. AARP; 2023 Apr 14 [cited 2025 Jun 12]. Available from: https://www.aarp.org/caregiving/medical/long-term-care-for-couples/
125. Kemp CL. Negotiating transitions in later life: married couples in assisted living. J Appl Gerontol. 2008 Jun;27(3):231–51. https://doi.org/10.1177/0733464807311656.
126. Pozzebon M, Douglas J, Ames D. Spouses' experience of living with a partner diagnosed with a dementia: a synthesis of the qualitative research. Int Psychogeriatr. 2016 Apr;28(4):537–56. https://doi.org/10.1017/S1041610215002239.
127. Frankowski AC, Clark LJ. Sexuality and intimacy in assisted living: residents' perspectives and experiences. Sex Res Social Policy. 2009 Dec;6(4):25–37. https://doi.org/10.1525/srsp.2009.6.4.25.
128. Tarzia L, Fetherstonhaugh D, Bauer M. Dementia, sexuality and consent in residential aged care facilities. J Med Ethics. 2012 Jun;38(1):609–13. https://doi.org/10.1136/medethics-2011-100453.
129. Sloane P. Sexual behavior in residents with dementia: guidelines explain how to respond. Contemporary Long-Term Care. 1993 Oct;66(69):108.
130. D'cruz M, Andrade C, Sathyanarayana Rao TS. The expression of intimacy and sexuality in persons with dementia. J Psychosexual Health. 2020 Jul;2(3–4):215–23. https://doi.org/10.1177/2631831820972859.
131. Bauer M, Fetherstonhaugh D, Tarzia L, Nay R, Wellman D, Beattie E. 'I always look under the bed for a man'. Needs and barriers to the expression of sexuality in residential aged care: the views of residents with and without dementia. Psychol Sex. 2012 Aug;4(3):296–309. https://doi.org/10.1080/19419899.2012.713869.
132. Simpson P, Wilson CB, Brown LJ, Dickinson T, Horne M. 'We've had our sex life way back': older care home residents, sexuality and intimacy. Ageing Soc. 2018 Jul;38(7):1478–501. https://doi.org/10.1017/S0144686X17000101.

133. Lindau ST, Dale W, Feldmeth G, Gavrilova N, Langa KM, Makelarski JA, Wroblewski K. Sexuality and cognitive status: a U.S. nationally representative study of home-dwelling older adults. J Am Geriatr Soc. 2018 Oct;66(10):1902–10. https://doi.org/10.1111/jgs.15511.
134. Rector S, Stiritz S, Morley JE. Sexuality, aging, and dementia. J Nutr Health Aging. 2020 Mar;24(4):366–70. https://doi.org/10.1007/s12603-020-1345-0.
135. Tabak N, Shemesh-Kigli R. Sexuality and Alzheimer's disease: can the two go together? Nurs Forum. 2006 Oct;41(4):158–66. https://doi.org/10.1111/j.1744-6198.2006.00054.x.
136. Abellard J, Rodgers C, Bales AL. Balancing sexual expression and risk of harm in elderly persons with dementia. J Am Acad Psychiatry Law. 2017 Dec;45(4):485–92.
137. Gayle BJ, Doll A. Sexuality & long-term care: understanding and supporting the needs of older adults. Soc Work Health Care. 2013 Jan;52(1):1–4. https://doi.org/10.1080/00981389.2012.728913.
138. Bartlett P. Sex, dementia, capacity and care homes. Liverp Law Rev. 2010 Oct;31(2):137–54. https://doi.org/10.1007/s10991-010-9077-6.
139. Lichtenberg PA, Strzepek DM. Assessments of institutionalized dementia patients' competencies to participate in intimate relationships. Gerontologist. 1990 Feb;30(1):117–20. https://doi.org/10.1093/geront/30.1.117.
140. Ho PJ, Goh YS. Health care professionals and care staff challenges and experiences of managing sexual expression among older adults ^{3}60 years in long-term care facilities: a qualitative review and meta-synthesis. Age Ageing. 2022 Jan;51(1):1–19. https://doi.org/10.1093/ageing/afab230.
141. Misaro J. Sexuality and dementia: assisted living staff negotiate the autonomy of residents' sexual needs [Dissertation]. ScholarWorks: Georgia State Univeristy; 2023. https://doi.org/10.57709/36387370.
142. Ward R, Vass AA, Aggarwal N, Garfield C, Cybyk B. A kiss is still a kiss?: the construction of sexuality in dementia care. Dementia. 2005 Feb;4(1):49–72. https://doi.org/10.1177/1471301205049190.

Chapter 6
Mental Health Care in Assisted Living

Cassandra L. Hua and Ijebusonma Agundu

Introduction

Individuals with mental health conditions are aging at unprecedented rates and are disproportionately represented in long-term care communities, including assisted living [1]. Mental health conditions, broadly defined by the Substance Abuse and Mental Health Services Administration, encompass a range of conditions that affect individuals' mood, behavior, and thinking. These conditions can range in severity from mild to serious mental illness that interferes with a person's life and ability to function [2]. This chapter focuses on the specific diagnoses of depression, anxiety disorders, bipolar disorder, and schizophrenia given their high prevalence in assisted living communities and the focus on these conditions in the long-term care literature [3]; however, it should be noted that mental health conditions encompass many more conditions (e.g., eating disorders, borderline personality disorder, posttraumatic stress disorder) that can affect individuals in assisted living communities just as they can in the general population [2].

Unfortunately, many assisted living communities may be unprepared to provide holistic, person-centered mental health care to the increasing number of assisted living residents with mental health conditions. Early models of assisted living were designed to provide supportive services (assistance) while maintaining the dignity, privacy, and choice of individuals as they age (living) [4]. However, as a whole, the assisted living sector evolved without the needs of this population in mind [1, 4]. This chapter explains the characteristics of each of the four conditions, provides context around the increase in mental health conditions in assisted living communities, and describes current treatment options. It also describes how assisted living

C. L. Hua (✉)
Department of Public Health, University of Massachusetts Lowell, Lowell, MA, USA
e-mail: Cassandra_hua@uml.edu

I. Agundu
Inpatient Psychiatry, Boston Children's Hospital, Waltham, MA, USA

H. Temkin-Greener and S. Zimmerman (eds.), *Assisted Living Through Research, Policy, and Practice*, https://doi.org/10.1007/978-3-032-32088-9_6

communities may currently fall short in promoting "assistance" and "living" for residents with mental health conditions, resulting in transitions to nursing homes. The chapter concludes by providing recommendations for research, practice, and policy and summarizing the points related to "assisted" and "living."

Depression. Depression is a diagnosis marked by symptoms that can negatively detract from quality of life such as diminished pleasure in activities, depressed mood, significant weight loss, insomnia, fatigue, and lessened ability to concentrate. Major depression is the most severe form of depression, while minor depression and dysthymia are less severe but still negatively impact quality of life [5]. Risk factors include female gender, chronic illness, cognitive and functional impairment, social isolation, and life transitions such as widowhood [5, 6]. The incidence of depression is not as high among older adults as it is among younger adults, yet some cases do appear first in later life [5]. In addition to impairing quality of life, depression is associated with suicide, self-neglect, loss of cognitive functioning, and all-cause mortality among older adults [5, 6]. The presence of subclinical depressive symptoms is associated with morbidities such as diabetes and premature mortality among older adults even in the absence of a formal diagnosis [6].

Anxiety disorder. Anxiety disorders encompass a broad range of conditions including social anxiety disorder, generalized anxiety disorder, agoraphobia, and panic disorder. Core symptoms include feelings of worry, fear, and nervousness and can also correspond with physical symptoms such as heart palpitations and muscle tension. Although some extent of anxiety is normal among individuals without anxiety disorders, anxiety disorders are differentiated by their intensity, severity, and the extent to which they impair social functioning [7]. In terms of presentation, women report higher rates of anxiety than men, and anxiety often co-occurs with depression. Although anxiety disorders usually first appear during childhood, anxiety disorders can also have a later life onset [7, 8]. Stressful life events, chronic health conditions, and lack of social contact are other risk factors among older adults [8].

Bipolar disorder. Bipolar disorder is a chronic mental health condition typically categorized into two types: bipolar I disorder and bipolar II disorder. Bipolar 1 is defined by the presence of at least one manic episode, marked by an abnormally elevated mood, increased activity or energy, and often accompanied by psychotic symptoms such as delusions of grandeur. These episodes can be severe enough to require hospitalization. Bipolar II disorder is characterized by recurrent hypomanic episodes combined with major depressive episodes. In hypomanic episodes, symptoms tend to last for shorter periods of time and without psychosis, and are milder than in manic episodes [9].

While bipolar I disorder affects men and women at similar rates, bipolar II disorder is more frequently diagnosed in women. The condition has a strong genetic component and typically emerges between the ages of 15 and 25, though it can be diagnosed later in life. Individuals with bipolar disorder often experience lifestyle challenges, including poor diet and smoking, which can increase the risk of cardiovascular disease. Additionally, the disorder is associated with a significantly higher risk of suicide [9].

Schizophrenia. Schizophrenia is one of the most serious mental health conditions and is characterized by reality distortion (hallucinations and delusions), disorganization (speech that is difficult to follow and disorganized behavior), and negative symptoms (blunted affect, lack of drive). Cognitive impairment is also now recognized as a key feature of schizophrenia [10]. The risk of schizophrenia is modestly higher in men than women and in terms of age, usually first occurs in the twenties; however, onset can occur past age 45 [10]. The heritability of the disorder is high. Schizophrenia can often cause poor occupational functioning and is associated with a shortened life expectancy. Although individuals with schizophrenia have a higher risk of suicide, much of the difference in life expectancy relates to differences in lifestyle factors (e.g., smoking, lack of activity, and poor diet). Despite these challenges, older adults with schizophrenia can still experience well-being and symptom improvement [10].

Increase in Prevalence and Characteristics of Residents with Mental Health Conditions in Assisted Living

Changes in public policy have, in part, been responsible for the increased presence of individuals with mental health conditions in assisted living, especially among those with more serious mental health conditions such as schizophrenia and bipolar disorder. Deinstitutionalization of state-run psychiatric hospitals became policy in the 1960s and 1970s in response to the inhumane conditions of some underfunded state hospitals and the new availability of antipsychotic medications in the outpatient setting [11]. Although the policy change was well-intentioned, there were not enough supportive services in the community to keep up with the increased demand. As a result, many individuals who had resided in state-run psychiatric institutions moved to nursing homes, and as explained below, also ultimately to assisted living. Today, individuals with serious mental health conditions continue to lack access to an adequate number of supportive services in the community as they age [3].

Previously, assisted living communities (separate from historic small "mom and pop" homes, which are often excluded from assisted living research) were unaffordable for individuals with mental health conditions largely because many are Medicaid recipients, and assisted living has traditionally served individuals who pay privately for their own care [4]. However, after the Olmstead vs. LC 1999 Supreme Court ruling, public entities were required to provide care to individuals with disabilities in the least restrictive setting possible [3, 11], and some states responded by reallocating Medicaid funding to home-and-community-based services such as assisted living waivers and assisted living state plans [12]. Therefore, the percent of individuals dually enrolled in Medicare and Medicaid has increased, including in assisted living; 17.5% of assisted living residents were dually enrolled in 2017 compared to 15.1% in 2013 [13, 14]. Given these changes in state policy, individuals with mental health conditions increasingly have access to assisted living communities, although Medicaid support is limited.

Research indicates that the prevalence of mental health conditions in assisted living is indeed increasing. In 2007, approximately 7.4% of fee-for-service Medicare beneficiaries in a national sample of residents in communities with at least 25 beds had a diagnosis of schizophrenia or bipolar disorder, compared to approximately 11.4% in 2017. This increase was faster than what was seen in the general community-residing population [1], indicating that the trend was not entirely the result of increased societal recognition of mental health conditions. The increase was also notable because it was seen in larger assisted living communities, which tend to have a lower prevalence of residents with mental health conditions than smaller assisted living communities [13].

Although the current prevalence of mental health conditions in assisted living varies depending on the criteria used to define mental health conditions and the method for how the study sample was constructed, the percent of individuals with mental health conditions in assisted living is believed to be high. According to the National Post-acute and Long-term Care Study, a nationally representative survey of long-term care providers, approximately 29% of assisted living residents had depression in 2020 [13]. This number is likely lower than what is reflected in reality, as prior research indicates that surveys likely underestimate the prevalence of chronic conditions such as depression due to reliance on the reports of staff who may not always know and document residents' medical conditions [15]. Additionally, direct care workers, who perform most of the personal care services in assisted living communities, often do not have training to perform formal assessments such as the Geriatric Depression Scale [16].

Studies that use Medicare administrative data have found a higher prevalence of depression in assisted living than what was found in the National Post-acute and Long-Term Care Study. Using claims data from the years 2018 and 2019, Temkin-Greener and colleagues found that 52% of residents had a diagnosis of depression, 11% had a diagnosis of bipolar disorder, and 16% had a diagnosis of schizophrenia in 2018 [17]. Another study using Medicare claims data found a prevalence of either anxiety or depression to be 66% in 2018 among a national cohort of assisted living residents [18]. An important caveat of many studies using Medicare data to study assisted living residents is that they exclude residents who are enrolled in Medicare Advantage because of previously incomplete chronic condition data for these residents. Additionally, residents with mental illness who are not age 65 and older or receiving Medicare benefits for a disability would not be captured [1, 17, 18].

There are also differences in the characteristics of residents who have mental health conditions when compared to those without mental health conditions. As implicated above, residents with schizophrenia and bipolar disorder are more likely to be younger than age 65; in 2017, approximately 64% of individuals with schizophrenia or bipolar disorder in a sample of assisted living residents were 65 and over compared to about 95% of residents without either condition [1]. Black and Hispanic assisted living residents are more likely to have diagnosed schizophrenia or bipolar disorder than White residents [1, 17], but there are less substantial racial differences in diagnosed depression and anxiety [17]. In addition, assisted living residents with schizophrenia and bipolar disorder are more likely to be dually eligible for Medicare and Medicaid and to qualify for Medicare due to having a disability compared to other assisted living residents [1, 17].

Residents with mental health conditions are also more likely to have comorbidities such as dementia. In 2018, approximately 63% of residents with a diagnosis of schizophrenia, bipolar disorder, or depression had dementia compared to 38% of individuals without one of these mental health conditions [17]. Diabetes, congestive heart failure, and chronic obstructive pulmonary disease are other comorbidities with a higher prevalence among individuals with mental health conditions [1, 17].

Further, there is substantial variability between and within states in the prevalence of mental health conditions in U.S. assisted living communities. For example, in 2017 the prevalence of schizophrenia and bipolar disorder ranged from 3.2% in Wyoming to 33.1% in New York; also, a mere 10% of assisted living communities had over half of the sample's assisted living residents with schizophrenia and bipolar disorder [1]. Differences in the distribution of individuals with mental health conditions in assisted living likely relate to differences in Medicaid reimbursement rates, differences in state policy, and market factors such as the availability of other residential care alternatives [1, 11]. Organizational factors likely also play a role, which can include litigation fears: as assisted living communities face an increasing number of lawsuits [19], some administrators may refuse to admit residents with mental health conditions.

The growing concentration of individuals with mental health conditions within a relatively small subset of assisted living communities is significant and may have far-reaching implications for care quality. Evidence from the nursing home literature shows that homes serving a high proportion of residents with serious mental illnesses—such as schizophrenia and bipolar disorder—tend to report poorer quality indicators, including lower staffing levels, reduced quality ratings, and a higher number of regulatory deficiency citations [20]. These disparities are often linked to strained resources, particularly in communities that are more dependent on Medicaid reimbursement, which typically provides lower payment rates than private pay sources [20]. A similar dynamic may be emerging in the assisted living sector.

Treatment and Management of Mental Health Conditions in Assisted Living Communities

Need for research trials on nonpharmacological treatments. Treatments can be broadly grouped into pharmacological (e.g., antidepressants such as selective serotonin reuptake inhibitors) and nonpharmacological (e.g., reminiscence therapy, exercise). Almost all research to date on the treatment of depression and anxiety in long-term care has been conducted in nursing homes [21–24]. Nonpharmacological treatments are generally found to be more effective than pharmacological treatments for nursing home residents with depression and anxiety, especially for residents with comorbid dementia [22, 24]. Systematic reviews of randomized controlled trials have found support for a diverse array of nonpharmacological interventions such as reminiscence therapy, exercise interventions, touch therapy, and companion animals. Music therapy has been found to be particularly effective in reducing anxiety among residents with and without dementia [23, 24]. For studies on both anxiety and depression, the studies have small sample sizes and have yet to be replicated in assisted living [21–24].

Most of the current literature on the treatment of bipolar disorder and schizophrenia has been conducted in community settings, largely ignoring residential long-term care [25–28]. Pharmacological treatments such as lithium and anticonvulsants can be beneficial for individuals with bipolar disorder but their safety and effectiveness vary based on medical comorbidities and residents' tolerance of side effects. To complicate matters, individuals with bipolar disorder often have difficulty adhering to medications [9]. Cognitive-behavioral therapy shows promise in clinical trials in improving symptoms and improving psychosocial functioning [25]. Lifestyle interventions, such as those that target sleep, smoking cessation, diet, and physical activity have been shown in randomized controlled trials to improve health habits and lower depressive symptoms among individuals with bipolar disorder [26].

Antipsychotics are the first line of treatment for schizophrenia, reducing symptoms such as delusions and improving social functioning. The drugs frequently, however, come with side effects such as substantial weight gain and sedation [10]. Psychosocial skills training interventions have been shown in randomized controlled trials to be effective in improving the functional and social skills of individuals with schizophrenia. These interventions teach everyday skills such as communication, organization, and financial management [27]. Other effective interventions promote skills in how to manage mental health and comorbid conditions simultaneously [27]. Physical activity interventions show promise in improving the symptoms of individuals with schizophrenia [28]. Work is needed to adapt interventions for schizophrenia and bipolar disorder for residential long-term care settings.

Need for specialized health and social services staff. There is a need for additional staff such as therapists, social workers, activity directors, and psychiatrists to provide care for assisted living residents with mental health conditions [30]. Data from the 2020 National Post-Acute and Long-Term Care Study indicate that 57% of assisted living communities offered on-site mental health services, while 51% provided access to social work services. Additionally, just over half (57%) employed a full-time activities director [13]. All of these roles are important for delivering nonpharmacological interventions [22, 24]. Qualitative research has documented persistent feelings of anxiety, depression, and social isolation among residents with mental health conditions, suggesting that existing services may be insufficient to meet residents' needs [29, 30].

Mental health services utilization is lower among assisted living communities with a high proportion of individuals who are dually eligible for Medicare and Medicaid [30]. One contributing factor is the low reimbursement rate provided by Medicaid, which may limit an assisted living community's ability to offer mental health services on site [20]. Additionally, low reimbursement rates could relate to staffing shortages and an inability to monitor residents for changes in mental health conditions or to arrange for mental health care visits [31]. Due to a lack of services on-site, many residents who need mental health care must seek the services outside of the assisted living community; unfortunately, finding mental health care outside of the community may be especially difficult for individuals with lower incomes, who may live in communities with fewer mental health resources and providers who are reluctant to accept Medicaid reimbursement [30].

The high prevalence of comorbidities among assisted living residents with mental health conditions presents additional challenges, particularly given the limited medical staffing requirements in these settings. Unlike nursing homes, assisted living communities are not federally mandated to employ licensed practical nurses (LPNs) or registered nurses (RNs) [4]. Still, according to the 2020 National Post-Acute and Long-Term Care Study, 43% of assisted living communities had a registered nurse on staff [13]. Medical services available in assisted living communities can vary widely, from basic tasks such as monitoring vital signs to more complex care, including the administration of intravenous medications [4]. While limiting on-site medical services may help keep assisted living more affordable compared to other long-term care options, inadequate access to skilled clinical oversight may increase the risk of complications, hospitalizations, or unnecessary transitions to higher levels of care [4].

Need for Staff Training on Mental Health Conditions. Research indicates that there is a lack of training among direct care workers in assisted living on how to best care for and interact with residents who have mental health conditions, especially those with disorders such as schizophrenia and bipolar disorder that can present with symptoms such as hallucinations or delusions [30]. In assisted living, many direct care staff have limited education beyond high school; they are also frequently assigned to many residents at one time given staffing shortages that are pervasive in the long-term care sector [4]. Staff have indicated that working with individuals who have schizophrenia and bipolar disorders can contribute to feelings of burnout [30, 32]. More so, residents with schizophrenia and bipolar disorder are often younger and physically stronger than the typical assisted living population, which can lead to heightened concern or fear among some staff members when aggressive or other behaviors arise [30].

Additional training may also help reduce the stigma toward individuals with mental health conditions that remain prevalent in assisted living environments—both among staff and fellow residents—mirroring broader societal biases [30]. This stigma can result in social isolation for affected individuals and may contribute to an underestimation of their capabilities [30]. When staff assume that residents with serious mental illness are less capable, it limits opportunities for meaningful engagement, effective treatment, and improvements in quality of life [30].

Additionally, direct care staff are not always able to differentiate between behaviors that express discomfort in persons with dementia and symptoms of psychotic disorders. This lack of recognition can also extend to managers [30]. Although there is some overlap between behaviors indicating discomfort in persons with dementia and behaviors related to mental health conditions such as schizophrenia, they are distinct conditions and require different treatment approaches. For example, long-term care residents with more severe mental illnesses often have them throughout their lives. However, after an acute episode, they may return to a baseline level of functioning with proper treatment. Conversely, individuals with dementia experience progressive cognitive decline [32].

Ability of Assisted Living Communities to Allow Aging in Place for Residents with Mental Health Conditions

Increased risk of nursing home transfer. Most older adults prefer to age in place, remaining in their homes or assisted living settings as their need for support increases, rather than moving to a nursing home-level of care [33]. Transfers to nursing homes can also be stigmatizing [35]. Prior research has demonstrated that assisted living residents who have mental health conditions are more likely to be transferred to a nursing home before the end of life than individuals without such conditions. For example, a study of 2,078 assisted living residents aged 65 and older across four states found that residents with depression experienced a 1.5 increase in the odds of transitioning to a nursing home than residents without depression [34]. Another state-specific study similarly found that individuals with a mental health condition were more likely to transition to a nursing home than residents without such diagnosis [36].

Although these studies were conducted over a decade ago, more recent evidence supports similar conclusions. A national cohort study involving 289,350 assisted living residents in 2018 and 2019 found that individuals diagnosed with depression had an elevated risk of nursing home transfer. Furthermore, residents diagnosed with both schizophrenia/bipolar disorder and dementia had a risk of nursing home placement that was twice the sample mean [17]. These findings raise some concerns about the ability of assisted communities to care for residents with mental health conditions.

Regulatory barriers in accessing care and/or remaining in assisted living. State regulations either enable or prevent residents with mental health conditions from aging in place in assisted living communities. Unlike in nursing homes, assisted living communities are regulated at the state level rather than the federal level. Within each state, different types of licenses define the scope of services that assisted living communities are permitted—or required—to provide, and they vary widely in their focus and requirements. In 2018, there were 350 different licenses and certifications that states used to govern assisted living. Some licenses follow more of a "housing model," emphasizing residential services with limited healthcare oversight—offering minimal support such as meal preparation, housekeeping, and basic supervision. Others align with a "medical model," requiring communities to provide more robust healthcare services, including licensed nursing staff, medication management, and regular health assessments [36]. Licenses that mandate higher levels of medical care may better support residents with mental health conditions given their high levels of comorbidity.

In addition to differences in service provision, state regulations also vary in terms of admission and retention policies for residents with mental health conditions. In nursing homes, the Nursing Home Reform Act of 1987 mandates a Pre-Admission Screening and Annual Resident Review (PASRR) to assess individuals for serious mental illness or intellectual disability prior to admission. Nursing homes are prohibited from admitting residents with mental health conditions unless they are equipped to provide appropriate mental health services. Although implementation challenges remain, the Act has been associated with improved quality of care in nursing homes [3].

By contrast, no equivalent federal law governs admissions to assisted living. Whether communities screen for mental health conditions, and whether such conditions can disqualify a person from admission or retention, is determined at the state level. As of 2018, about 54% of assisted living communities operated under licenses that restricted admission based on the presence of a mental health condition—either alone or alongside other factors, such as physical health limitations [37].

Some states, however, have adopted more supportive regulatory frameworks to promote aging in place for individuals with mental health needs. For example, Florida's Limited Mental Health (LMH) license requires assisted living communities to provide not only basic services but also case management and at least 6 h of mental health training for direct care staff. Other licensing structures do not mandate on-site mental health services but still require that residents have access to appropriate mental healthcare through community-based providers [17].

Research, Policy, and Practice Recommendations

Investment is needed to fund trials on nonpharmacological interventions in the assisted living setting that are designed to treat symptoms of mental health conditions. Even when pharmacological treatments are deemed important, such as in schizophrenia, treatment can be enhanced by interventions such as social skills training [27]. Yet, we know very little about what works even in the nursing home (where there has been more research) due to small sample sizes, lack of staff fidelity to the intervention, and heterogeneity in methodological approaches [21–24]. The extant research has also focused on depression and anxiety and has largely ignored schizophrenia and bipolar disorder [21–24]. Even if the nursing home literature were complete, assisted living has unique features such as a lack of registered nurse presence and a more home-like setting that could cause the effectiveness of treatments to be different than what is seen in nursing homes [4]. Thus, research into effective interventions in the assisted living setting is needed.

State regulations to assess the presence of mental health conditions at admission to assisted living communities should be commonplace. Routine assessment of mental health conditions upon admission is critical because untreated mental health conditions among older adults are associated with a range of adverse outcomes, including diminished quality of life, functional decline, accelerated cognitive impairment, increased risk of hospitalization, and even premature mortality [6]. By identifying mental health conditions early, assisted living communities can develop individualized care or service plans that better address residents' psychological and emotional well-being, in addition to their physical needs. Moreover, a standardized mental health assessment can help determine whether a community is an appropriate setting for a prospective resident or if their care needs exceed the assisted living community's capabilities. This process may help reduce the likelihood of premature transfers to more restrictive environments such as nursing homes and help ensure that residents receive services aligned with their overall needs [37].

Mental health training for direct care staff is needed. As the proportion of residents in assisted living communities with mental health conditions continues to grow, it is essential that staff are equipped to recognize, understand, and effectively communicate with individuals who have these conditions. A Delphi panel of 19 experts in long-term care voiced that staff training in mental health care was of high-quality importance to providing high-quality care in assisted living and that doing so was perceived as feasible [39].

Few examples of training interventions in the literature exist that are specific to mental health in long-term care, but extant studies indicate that such interventions can potentially be effective at improving direct care worker knowledge. For example, a two-to-three-hour web-based online training program for direct care workers called CARES® Serious Mental Illness™ (CARES SMI; a modification of the CARES® Approach framework used for people with dementia) focuses on teaching staff how to respond to residents using a person-centered approach, making sure that residents' emotional needs are met. Pilot work indicates that the CARES SMI web-based training is feasible and acceptable to direct care workers in nursing homes and assisted living communities. Direct care staff also report increased knowledge and confidence in working with residents with mental health conditions. However, the training has yet to be tested on a larger scale [32].

Telehealth may play a role in improving access to on-site care. Providing access to adequate mental health services in assisted living communities is essential but often difficult to achieve given current staff shortages and affordability concerns. The Delphi panel of long-term care experts ranked the provision of on-site mental health care as very important for quality of life and care outcomes, but also identified it as having low feasibility under current conditions [39].

Telehealth may help expand mental health services, such as counseling and psychiatric services, to residents who live in an assisted living community with little in-house service provision of mental health care. Telehealth use became more commonplace after the COVID-19 pandemic due to restrictions on in-person visits and Medicare's expansion of telehealth coverage. Previous work found that quarterly mental health telehealth utilization among a national sample of assisted living residents with dementia increased after the COVID-19 pandemic, from 0.4% to 6.2%. Although the use decreased somewhat in the last quarters of 2020 (to 4.6%), it did not return to baseline levels. Encouragingly, telehealth did not appear to increase racial, ethnic, or socioeconomic disparities in mental healthcare utilization [31].

Research on the effectiveness of mental health telehealth in long-term care is scarce. An integrated review of 16 studies of telehealth delivered in the nursing home setting for various services (e.g., psychiatry, geriatric care) found that telehealth use was generally accepted by providers and families, who believed that telehealth increased the speed at which residents could access care. Further, there was some preliminary evidence that telehealth can help reduce emergency department visits and hospitalizations. However, the studies were methodologically heterogeneous and the samples were small and nongeneralizable [40]. Even less has been published on the effectiveness of mental telehealth in assisted living, a setting with unique opportunities and challenges. On one hand, the lack of medical presence in assisted living could make accessibility of telehealth methodology even more important, but on the other hand, there may be a lack of staff available to implement a telehealth program [3].

Implications for "Assisted" and "Living"

The prevalence of mental health conditions is notable and rising among residents in assisted living communities. In some ways, this trend reflects progress: expanded funding for Medicaid home-and-community-based service waivers and similar policy changes have improved access to assisted living for individuals with behavioral health needs, allowing more people to receive care in less restrictive, presumably more person-centered settings. Assisted living's philosophical emphasis on a "home-like" environment—prioritizing autonomy, dignity, and choice—holds particular promise for individuals with mental health conditions who need support but do not require the intensity of services provided in nursing homes. This philosophy embodies the "living" component of assisted living.

At present, however, most assisted living communities lack the resources necessary to provide sufficient assistance—the other critical component of assisted living—for a growing population of residents with mental health conditions. There is a lack of tested nonpharmacological approaches to manage symptoms, insufficient staff training, and a lack of holistic mental health care services on-site. Assisted living residents with mental health conditions are more likely to be transferred to a nursing home at the end of life, underscoring the inability of residents to age in place. To address these challenges, new and innovative strategies are needed. These strategies include testing evidence-based interventions, increasing staff training opportunities, improving mental health screening and care planning processes, and leveraging technologies such as telehealth to extend the reach of behavioral health professionals.

Competing Interests The authors have no conflicts of interest to declare that are relevant to the content of this chapter.

References

1. Hua CL, Cornell PY, Zimmerman S, Winfree J, Thomas KS. Trends in serious mental illness in US assisted living compared to nursing homes and the community: 2007–2017. Am J Geriatr Psychiatry. 2021;29(5):434–44.
2. Substance Abuse and Mental Health Administration. Mental Health [Internet]. Available from: https://www.samhsa.gov/mental-health
3. Bucy T, Moeller K, Bowblis JR, Shippee N, Fashaw-Walters S, Winkelman T, Shippee T. Serious mental illness in the nursing home literature: a scoping review. Gerontol Geriatr Med. 2022;8:23337214221101260.
4. Zimmerman S, Stone R, Carder P, Thomas K. Does assisted living provide assistance and promote living? Health Aff (Millwood). 2024;43(5):674–81.
5. Casey DA. Depression in older adults: a treatable medical condition. Prim Care. 2017;44(3):499–510.
6. Fiske A, Wetherell JL, Gatz M. Depression in older adults. Annu Rev Clin Psychol. 2009;5(1):363–89.
7. Penninx BW, Pine DS, Holmes EA, Reif A. Anxiety disorders [published correction appears in Lancet. 2021 Mar 6;397(10277):880. Lancet. 2021;397(10277):914–927.
8. Vink D, Aartsen MJ, Schoevers RA. Risk factors for anxiety and depression in the elderly: a review. J Affect Disord. 2008;106(1–2):29–44.
9. Nierenberg AA, Agustini B, Köhler-Forsberg O, Cusin C, Katz D, Sylvia LG, Peters A, Berk M. Diagnosis and treatment of bipolar disorder: a review. JAMA. 2023;330(14):1370–80.
10. Jauhar S, Johnstone M, McKenna PJ. Schizophrenia. Lancet. 2022;399(10323):473–86.
11. Ng T, Stone J, Harrington C. Medicaid home and community-based services: how consumer access is restricted by state policies. J Aging Soc Policy. 2015;27(1):21–46.
12. Cornell PY, Hua C, Rahman M, Gadkari G, Gunderson R, Smith L, Thomas KS. Association of Medicaid financing and concentration of assisted living residents dually eligible for Medicare and Medicaid. JAMA Health Forum 2023;4(2):e225338.
13. National Center for Health Statistics. Data from the 2020 national post-acute and long-term care study. https://www-cdcgov.revproxy.brown.edu/nchs/npals/webtables/overview.html, Accessed 25th Sep 2024.
14. Harris-Kojetin L, Sengupta M, Park-Lee E, et al. Long-term care providers and services users in the United States: data from the national Study of long-term care providers, 2013–2014. Vital Health Stat. 2016;3(38):1–105.
15. Zimmerman S, Guo W, Mao Y, Li Y, Temkin-Greener H. Health care needs in assisted living: survey data may underestimate chronic conditions. J Am Med Dir Assoc. 2021;22(2):471–3.
16. Brühl KG, Luijendijk HJ, Muller MT. Nurses' and nursing assistants' recognition of depression in elderly who depend on long-term care. J Am Med Dir Assoc. 2007;8(7):441–5.
17. Temkin-Greener H, Guo W, McGarry B, Cai S. Serious mental illness in assisted living communities: association with nursing home placement. J Am Med Dir Assoc. 2024;25(5):917–22.
18. Temkin-Greener H, Mao Y, McGarry B, Zimmerman S, Li Y. Health care use and outcomes in assisted living communities: race, ethnicity, and dual eligibility. Med Care Res Rev. 2022;79(4):500–10.
19. Fetterolf M, Kao P, Castle N. Rise in assisted living lawsuits indicates the need for a consumer-centered model of care. JHNR. 2019;2019(5):24–6.
20. Jester DJ, Hyer K, Bowblis JR. Quality concerns in nursing homes that serve large proportions of residents with serious mental illness. Gerontologist. 2020;60(7):1312–21.

21. Simning A, Simons KV. Treatment of depression in nursing home residents without significant cognitive impairment: a systematic review. Int Psychogeriatr. 2017;29(2):209–26.
22. Watt JA, Goodarzi Z, Veroniki AA, Nincic V, Khan PA, Ghassemi M, Lai Y, Treister V, Thompson Y, Schneider R, Tricco AC, Straus SE. Comparative efficacy of interventions for reducing symptoms of depression in people with dementia: systematic review and network meta-analysis. BMJ. 2021 Mar 24;372:n532.
23. Atchison K, Watt JA, Ewert D, Toohey AM, Ismail Z, Goodarzi Z. Non-pharmacologic and pharmacologic treatments for anxiety in long-term care: a systematic review and meta-analysis. Age Ageing 2022 Sep 2;51(9):afac195.
24. Brown Wilson C, Arendt L, Nguyen M, Scott TL, Neville CC, Pachana NA. Nonpharmacological interventions for anxiety and dementia in nursing homes: a systematic review. Gerontologist. 2019;59(6):e731–42.
25. Chiang KJ, Tsai JC, Liu D, Lin CH, Chiu HL, Chou KR. Efficacy of cognitive-behavioral therapy in patients with bipolar disorder: a meta-analysis of randomized controlled trials. PLoS ONE. 2017 May 4;12(5):e0176849.
26. Simjanoski M, Patel S, Boni R, Balanzá-Martínez V, Frey BN, Minuzzi L, Kapczinski F, Cardoso TA. Lifestyle interventions for bipolar disorders: a systematic review and meta-analysis. Neurosci Biobehav Rev. 2023 Sept;152:105257.
27. Bartels SJ, DiMilia PR, Fortuna KL, Naslund JA. Integrated care for older adults with serious mental illness and medical comorbidity: evidence-based models and future research directions. Clin Geriatr Med. 2020;36(2):341–52.
28. Rosenbaum S, Tiedemann A, Sherrington C, Curtis J, Ward PB. Physical activity interventions for people with mental illness: a systematic review and meta-analysis. J Clin Psychiatry. 2014;75(9):964–74.
29. David D, Lassell RKF, Mazor M, Brody AA, Schulman-Green D. "I have a lotta sad feelin'" - unaddressed mental health needs and self-support strategies in Medicaid-funded assisted living. J Am Med Dir Assoc. 2023;24(6):833–40.
30. Morgan LA, Perez R, Frankowski AC, Nemec M, Bennett CR. Mental illness in assisted living: challenges for quality of life and care. J Hous Elderly. 2016;30(2):185–98.
31. Temkin-Greener H, Hua Y, Cai S. Assisted living residents with dementia: disparities in mental health services pre and during COVID-19. J Am Geriatr Soc. 2024;72(6):1760–9.
32. Molinari V, Hobday JV, Roker R, Kunik ME, Kane R, Kaas MJ, Mehrotra C, Williams CL, Robbins JC, Dobbs D. Impact of serious mental illness online training for certified nursing assistants in long term care. Gerontol Geriatr Educ. 2017;38(4):359–74.
33. Davis MR. Despite pandemic, percentage of older adults who want to age in place stays steady [Internet]. 2021 Nov 18. Available from: https://www.aarp.org/home-family/your-home/info-2021/home-and-community-preferences-survey.html
34. Watson LC, Garrett JM, Sloane PD, Gruber-Baldini AL, Zimmerman S. Depression in assisted living: results from a four-state study. Am J Geriatr Psychiatry. 2003;11(5):534–42.
35. Zimmerman S, Dobbs D, Roth EG, Goldman S, Peeples AD, Wallace B. Promoting and protecting against stigma in assisted living and nursing homes. Gerontologist. 2016;56(3):535–47.
36. Dobbs D, Hayes J, Chapin R, Oslund P. The relationship between psychiatric disorders and the ability to age in place in assisted living. Am J Geriatr Psychiatry. 2006;14(7):613–20.
37. Smith L, Carder P, Hua C, Zimmerman S, Sloane PD, Zhang W, Wretman CJ, Cornell P, Thomas KS. A national typology of health service regulation in assisted living. Gerontologist 2024 May 1;64(5):gnad109.
38. Kaskie B, Xu L, Smith L, Bounds D, Carder P, Thomas KS. Pathways into assisted living communities: admission limitations and assessment requirements across the United States. J Am Med Dir Assoc. 2023;24(6):821–6.
39. Zimmerman S, Sloane PD, Wretman CJ, Cao K, Silbersack J, Carder P, Thomas KS, Allen J, Butrum K, Chicotel T, Giorgio P, Hernandez M, Kales H, Katz P, Klinger JH, Kunze M, Laxton C, McNealley V, Meeks S, O'Neil K, Pace D, Resnick B, Schwartz L, Seitz D, Smetanka L, Van Haitsma K. Recommendations for medical and mental health care in assisted living based

on an expert Delphi consensus panel: a consensus statement. JAMA Netw Open. 2022 Sep 1;5(9):e2233872.
40. Groom LL, McCarthy MM, Stimpfel AW, Brody AA. Telemedicine and telehealth in nursing homes: an integrative review. J Am Med Dir Assoc. 2021;22(9):1784–801.

Chapter 7
Medical Care in Assisted Living

Sarah Howd and Thomas Caprio

Introduction

Assisted living has become a cornerstone of community based residential care in the United States, offering an alternative to traditional institutional care for older adults who require support with activities of daily living but wish to maintain as much independence as possible. Originally envisioned as a non-medical, socially supportive environment, the reality of today's communities reflects a growing demand to care for residents with complex medical, cognitive, and behavioral needs. As residents live longer and with more chronic conditions, the boundaries between assisted living and skilled nursing care have become increasingly blurred. This chapter explores the evolving role of medical care in assisted living, including the regulatory landscape, staffing models, clinical challenges, and opportunities for policy innovation. It aims to provide healthcare professionals and policymakers with a deeper understanding of how medical services are delivered in assisted living communities and how these services influence resident outcomes, care transitions, and the broader health system.

S. Howd
University of Rochester Medicine Geriatrics Group Senior Living Practice, Department of Medicine, School of Medicine and Dentistry, University of Rochester, Rochester, NY, USA
e-mail: Sarah_Howd@urmc.rochester.edu

T. Caprio (✉)
Department of Medicine, School of Medicine and Dentistry, Home Healthcare and Hospice, University of Rochester, Rochester, NY, USA
e-mail: Thomas_Caprio@urmc.rochester.edu

H. Temkin-Greener and S. Zimmerman (eds.), *Assisted Living Through Research, Policy, and Practice*, https://doi.org/10.1007/978-3-032-32088-9_7

Importance of Understanding Assisted Living Licensing

Assisted living communities are licensed, based on state regulations, to serve a broad spectrum of residents, aiming to support aging in place ("living") as care needs change over time. Three different levels of ("assisted") services may be offered by assisted living communities, often categorized as traditional, enhanced, and special needs, based on the residents' care requirements.

The traditional assisted living community is meant for people who are mostly independent but need help with basic activities of daily living, such as bathing, dressing, and grooming. Residents may receive assistance with medication management, housekeeping, transportation, and social activities, but should not need complex medical care or continuous nursing supervision. Some communities have developed an "a la carte" approach where a resident's monthly cost is based on basic room and board services and specifically on personal care they require, for example how much assistance they need with dressing or how frequently they need medications dispensed.

Enhanced assisted living offers a higher level of support for residents with more significant physical or health-related needs. In addition to standard assistance with activities of daily living, enhanced care may include help with ambulation and transfers, complex medication management (such as insulin injections), and management of durable medical equipment (like oxygen or catheters). These residents often have chronic conditions that require closer monitoring and might otherwise need nursing home placement without this level of support.

Special needs assisted living commonly refers to memory care and is designed for residents with dementia or other cognitive disorders. These units are typically secured to prevent wandering and are staffed by personnel with extra training in dementia care. Services emphasize structure, routine, and safety, while supporting residents' behavioral and emotional needs with a higher staff-to-resident ratio.

Care in assisted living is primarily funded out-of-pocket, but may also be covered, at least in part, by private long-term care insurance. The mean cost of assisted living in the United States is nearly $4,500 per month, or about $54,000 per year [1]. However, the median cost is somewhat higher, over $6,200 per month, translating to roughly $74,000 annually [2]. These figures reflect typical pricing for standard assisted living services, though costs vary significantly by location, level of care, and amenities offered.

Aging in Place and "Acuity Creep"

Adults over age 65 comprise the sector of the population with the most rapid growth in the United States. This has led to increased need for long-term residential care options and assisted living communities have been expanding to suit this need. Assisted living communities are less expensive and less institutional than nursing homes and are perceived to provide more supportive care than independent living, making them an appealing option for those no longer able to live independently [3].

When a resident moves into assisted living, they may expect this to be their "forever" home where they will age in place for as long as possible. Aging in place benefits the residents as well as the assisted living providers. However, the median length of stay in assisted living is estimated to be 22 months, so in reality these communities often offer a temporary home until care needs dictate the necessity for an individual to move to a higher level of care (i.e., nursing home) [2]. The National Center for Assisted Living estimates that around 60% of assisted living residents eventually move to skilled nursing facilities [2]. One study, using Medicare data, examined the cohort of assisted living residents who died in 2016 and found that about 57% died in the assisted living, and the remainder died in nursing homes or hospitals [4]. Both assisted living providers and residents feel the tension of balancing the desire to age in place with managing increased care requirements [5]. Criteria for determining how long a resident can age in place are often unclear, and inconsistencies in "move out" policies may lead to inequity and injustice to the resident. This may also lead to anxiety about potentially being forced to move at some point, as nursing homes are often considered places of "last resort" [6].

Research indicates that families play a significant role in decisions regarding the care and placement of older adults in long-term residential care settings. Studies have shown that family involvement is crucial in transfer decisions, with families often influencing the timing and necessity of transitions to higher levels of care. The absence of advance directives and family preferences has been identified as factors contributing to decisions to keep residents in assisted living rather than moving them to skilled nursing facilities. Thus, families may be able to influence assisted living communities to maintain residents in place, especially when they perceive that the current setting meets the individual's needs [7, 8]. However, if assisted living is providing more care than it is licensed to and the resident has a poor outcome, they can be held legally responsible.

The cognitive and physical status of an assisted living resident will change over time, and regular communication with family becomes critically important in making them aware of how care plans can adapt to these changes, and if the needs of the resident are starting to exceed the services that the community can provide. In communities licensed to provide enhanced care, a resident may be more likely to extend their length of stay if they receive help with activities of daily living such as ambulation and toileting or with medical management of oxygen or catheters. To successfully care for residents on enhanced care, communities must enact policies and procedures for providing the higher level of care and assuring that their staffing levels and training meet these enhanced requirements, which usually means employing more nurses to provide the care. Agreeing to provide enhanced care without deploying appropriate resources opens communities to significant legal risk. In many states, medical providers must complete a resident assessment, on admission and annually, to determine whether the resident is medically and mentally suited for assisted living and does not have continuous skilled nursing care needs. Thus, medical providers must have a solid understanding of how much care assisted living can provide. If these standards are not met, the assisted living community needs to work with the family to pursue a higher level of care.

Physician Perspective on Caring for Assisted Living Residents

Assisted living communities were designed to provide personal care and social supports to their residents to facilitate "aging in place." But as the residents' medical complexity and physical frailty increases, the attainment of this goal and the provision of person-centered care increasingly require the coordinated involvement of physicians, nurse practitioners, and physician assistants, together with the assisted living staff of nurses, direct care workers, and case managers when available [9]. A survey of 165 physicians who had patients in 125 assisted living communities across 27 states found that on average, physicians were only "somewhat confident" in the assisted living staff's ability to provide appropriate care, though trust was higher when there was a nursing presence on site [10]. This lack of confidence in staff ability to monitor or support a resident with an acute medical issue may also be evident in the substantially higher emergency department (ED) transfer rates, compared to those among the nursing home residents [11].

With the great amount of variability in the services offered to assisted living residents in different communities, medical providers caring for these older adults need to understand, in broad strokes, the licensing and state regulations affecting the delivery of services to their patients. This knowledge allows the medical providers to utilize the services of the assisted living to optimize the care of their patients. For example, if the staff of an assisted living is able to check a resident's blood pressure, following a medication change, a medical provider can order blood pressure checks with proper call parameters, for a discrete amount of time, to evaluate whether the change was effective. If a patient with cognitive impairment needs to start wearing oxygen overnight, and they live in an assisted living that offers enhanced services providing reminders and assistance with placing the oxygen, that important facet of their medical care becomes much more achievable.

Studies have explored physicians' roles in assisted living communities highlighting that they often play a limited and indirect role in these settings, relying heavily on staff for communication and resident updates. Dys et al., called for clearer role definitions, improved care coordination, and better integration of physicians into assisted living teams to support residents' complex health needs, emphasizing the importance of policy and practice changes to enhance physician involvement and improve resident outcomes [12].

Impacts on the Health Care System

Older adults residing in assisted living can have a significant impact on the local health system. Assisted living staff are often not licensed to perform clinical assessments, but prior to a resident being admitted or readmitted, they may complete pre-admission questionnaires and review physician or nurse evaluations; in states requiring a registered nurse, the clinical assessment can be conducted by the nurse. Once a resident has moved in, staff become responsible for observing changes in conditions and for reporting them to the medical provider and the resident's family, and for seeking the appropriate medical evaluation. As in most communities staff are not permitted to clinically assess residents, this often leads to utilizing emergency responders and/or the ED to provide that assessment. This comes with significant risk, since older adults are likely to experience a functional decline and a higher rate of poor outcomes after ED discharge [13, 14]. Assisted living communities are high utilizers of emergency departments, with studies estimating that over one-third of all residents will present to the ED in a year [15]. ED visits are more costly for adults over age 65, averaging $1,110 for treat-and-release scenarios, so there is a substantial financial implication of frequent ED utilization [16]. Even proximity to an ED can impact the rate of its use, with assisted living residents living closer to an ED being more likely to have a visit. Though residents living closer to ED had higher rates of visits, they had similar rates of hospital admissions to those living further away, suggesting that many were being evaluated in the ED for non-urgent care [17].

Not only is it important for primary care providers to understand the services their patients receive in assisted living, but it is also imperative that hospital teams caring for patients admitted from assisted living know this as well. The ability to discharge a patient back to their community depends on the return to the baseline level of functioning, or if that is not attainable, the capacity of the assisted living to provide the amount of care needed post-discharge (especially after an acute illness). Residents from traditional assisted living communities may need to prove their ability to be independent with mobility and personal care to return to their community. If this is not possible, a stay in a skilled nursing facility for rehabilitation or long-term care may be necessary. If the resident is from an assisted living with enhanced services, they may be able to return back with more hands-on support for mobility or management of medical equipment like a catheter or oxygen. Enhanced care comes with extra cost to the resident, so this needs to be financially feasible as well. In our experience, assisted living communities often request that the resident is assessed visually by their staff before accepting them back, and coordinating these evaluations may lengthen the stay in the hospital. Many times assisted living will not be as well-staffed on the weekends and may refuse to accept a hospitalized resident back on a Saturday or a Sunday, so the risk of hospital-acquired complications may rise for these residents. Communication between the hospital team, including nursing, social work, and medical providers with the assisted living staff, resident's family, and their primary medical team is critical to ensure successful transitions between different levels of care.

Nursing Roles in Assisted Living

Nursing roles in assisted living vary from state to state, and even from community to community within the same state. States have specific regulations regarding nursing service requirements. There are 34 states which require assisted living communities to have registered nurses (RN); half mandating RNs as part of the direct care staff, and the other half requiring RNs to be available for consultation for issues like directing the use of as needed medications for residents who are not cognitively able to report symptoms and request a treatment [18]. State regulatory agencies may allow communities to retain residents with temporary skilled nursing care needs to be cared for by their licensed nurse staff or a home care agency [19]. However, in some states, for example in New York, when a resident has continued skilled nursing needs a resident may be deemed unable to stay in assisted living. State regulations generally allow nurses in assisted living to report a change in condition but not provide a clinical assessment of the situation, which must be performed by a physician, nurse practitioner, or physician assistant.

There is growing research evidence that state regulations requiring licensed nursing staff in assisted living are positively associated with better resident outcomes. When ED utilization of assisted living residents was examined, states that did not have a requirement for nursing in assisted living were found to have the highest rates of ED visits in the country [15]. A multi-state longitudinal study of nearly 1,900 assisted living residents found that communities with a higher proportion of licensed nursing staff had significantly lower hospitalization rates, particularly as dementia prevalence increased. These findings indicate that greater nursing presence in assisted living improves resident health outcomes and may reduce the need for acute care [20].

Nurses are also critically important in proper medication management in assisted living, which is one of the most common services provided in this care setting. A large, nationwide study of assisted living and its residents' characteristics noted that staff provided oversight and cuing of medications for 92% of the residents [21]. In a study of state-level regulations of assisted living communities, Temkin-Greener et al., identified significant differences in the stringency of regulations focused on medication management and licensed nursing staff [22]. Another study showed positive associations between administration of injected medications by licensed nurses and residents' outcomes at the end of life, specifically fewer burdensome transitions to acute settings [23].

Home health agencies play a vital role in extending the capacity of assisted living communities to provide medical and rehabilitative services. Because most assisted living communities are not licensed or staffed to provide continuous skilled nursing services, they often rely on external home health providers to deliver short-term or intermittent skilled care or rehabilitation as ordered by a medical provider. This includes skilled nursing for wound care, medication management, catheter care, and injections, as well as rehabilitative therapies such as physical therapy, occupational therapy, and speech-language pathology. Rehabilitative therapy interventions can influence resident safety and continued residence by improving strength, mobility, and the ability to complete personal care tasks. Communication between agency clinicians and assisted living staff is paramount to ensuring appropriate implementation of the home health plan of care. Variability in state regulations and the capacity of assisted living communities to accommodate frequent clinical monitoring may limit the implementation of certain interventions. Medical providers must assess whether a resident's care needs can be safely supported through a combination of assisted living services and home health clinicians.

Medical Visits on Site in the Assisted Living

In the previously mentioned physician survey, fewer than half reported seeing patients on site in their assisted living community [10]. With the increasing frailty among assisted living residents, most with multiple co-morbidities [20], many are fully dependent on transportation services to attend medical appointments in a clinic. Taking the resident out of their home setting reduces the amount of collateral information available to the medical provider from assisted living staff who provide the day-to-day care. Up to 70% of assisted living residents have some level of cognitive impairment, and 44% are diagnosed with dementia [24], so in many cases the medical decision-making capacity of a resident is diminished. This requires family or support people to be engaged in medical care planning with the primary care provider, who in turn needs to coordinate a resident's individualized care with assisted living staff members. Providing medical services for acute and chronic issues for assisted living residents is often complex. Much communication is conducted over the phone, and depending on state regulations, extra paperwork may need to be completed by the medical provider and written orders and faxes may need to be reviewed, for example addressing weight changes, missed medications, and order clarifications. Research into innovative ways to deliver medical care on site to assisted living residents is critical as it pertains not only to the older adult's ability to age in place, but may also impact the local health system, such as the high rate of ED utilization that has been previously mentioned.

The acceptance of telemedicine as a method to evaluate and manage patients expanded greatly during the COVID-19 pandemic, with the Centers for Medicare and Medicaid Services (CMS) solidifying a payment model for the service. Though the use of telemedicine for regular visits or chronic health checkups may be restricted in terms of reimbursement in the future, the utility of video visits for urgent evaluations of patients where they reside is anticipated to remain sustainable. A study conducted prior to COVID-19 pandemic, showed that telemedicine visits in senior living facilities (independent and assisted living) reduced the yearly frequency of ED visits by 24% [25]. Telemedicine evaluations satisfy the regulations for medical assessment for change in condition, and if offered by the medical provider in an efficient manner, can establish a treatment in place plan for the resident and may prevent a call to 911 and a trip to the ED.

Medical Direction in Assisted Living

Unlike nursing homes, there is no mandate for assisted living communities to have a medical provider in the role of medical director. However, there are instances where state regulations require assisted living communities to formalize a relationship with a medical provider for different purposes. For example, the New York State Department of Health requires assisted living to have a physician or nurse practitioner signed on as the laboratory director in order to obtain a limited-service laboratory registration, allowing assisted living staff to perform such testing as blood glucose readings or viral swab testing. Medical providers should not take on this role without a clear understanding of how assisted living communities are regulated and operated, which a medical director would have. As a result of increased knowledge of how the assisted living operates, physicians serving as medical directors of an assisted living community were consistently more confident in the AL staff's capabilities [10]. Because assisted living communities operate in such a heterogeneous way, the role of a medical director can be tailored to the needs of the community. Examples of services a medical director can offer an assisted living community include round-the-clock availability for urgent facility issues, review of policies and procedures, participation in quality assurance and process improvement, provision of emergency treatment, assistance in transfers of care, offering staff in-service education, and serving as laboratory director [26]. In 2022, Zimmerman et al., conducted a Delphi consensus study with 19 national experts to establish recommendations for medical and mental health care in assisted living, identifying 43 key practices spanning staff training, nursing services, resident assessment, care planning, policies, and clinician involvement. Recommendations pertaining to medical oversight included all assisted living residents having a primary care provider to lead general medical management and provide baseline and ongoing health assessments. The primary care provider should have a consistent and standardized communication process with the assisted living staff and be part of the interdisciplinary team along with nurses, administrators, social workers, and direct care workers [27]. Medical directors can be integral to training assisted living nursing and direct care staff, offering ongoing education in geriatric syndromes, behavioral and mental health care, and infection control.

The COVID-19 pandemic brought to light the lack of general understanding of the assisted living setting from both federal and state government and regional health systems. Despite assisted living being the largest provider of residential care in the country, initial national directives from the Centers of Disease Control and Prevention to mitigate and manage COVID-19 outbreaks excluded this important sector of residential long-term care [28]. Instructions were given to nursing homes and to senior independent living communities, leaving assisted living communities to decide which guidance to follow. The variability in resulting assisted living policies made it especially difficult for primary care providers to implement measures to provide best care for assisted living residents in preventing and treating infections. In our experience, as contracted medical directors of several assisted living communities in the Rochester, New York area, we were able to implement policies facility-wide to provide appropriate monitoring of infected or exposed individuals in their home setting, often preventing hospital transfers and limiting spread of COVID-19 within the building. As medical directors, we are able to help guide administrators in management of visitation policies and assist in communication to residents and their families. Medical directors ordered and oversaw viral testing for any resident or staff within the community, and when COVID-19 vaccines became available, they were able to quickly and effectively provide vaccinations to all in the assisted living community.

The Post-Acute and Long-Term Care Medical Association (PALTMed) has been instrumental in advancing the role of medical providers in assisted living. Recognizing the increasing clinical complexity of assisted living residents, PALTMed has promoted the importance of the interdisciplinary team (IDT) in delivering coordinated, person-centered care that integrates medical, nursing, and psychosocial support. Over the past five years, PALTMed's national meetings have included multiple assisted living-focused presentations addressing models of care, medical oversight, and best practices [29]. In response to requests from providers nationwide, PALTMed also developed a sample medical direction contract to serve as a resource for expanding structured medical practice within assisted living communities [30]. These initiatives reflect PALTMed's commitment to strengthening the presence and effectiveness of medical professionals and IDTs in assisted living.

Advance Directives and End-of-Life Care

Advance care planning is a critical yet complex aspect of medical care in assisted living. While most residents enter assisted living with the hope of aging in place, many communities face regulatory and logistical barriers that affect their ability to support residents through end of life. State regulations, liability concerns, and staffing limitations all shape what services can be delivered as residents decline.

In many communities, corporate policies prohibit staff from initiating cardiopulmonary resuscitation (CPR) due to the inability to guarantee 24/7 availability of trained responders. This often surprises families, who may assume that staff can intervene during a medical emergency. In 2013, a senior living community in California received negative publicity when staff called 911 for a resident who had collapsed and then refused to start performing CPR despite the 911 operator's instructions, citing the facility policy not to do so [31]. In the end, the family was supportive of the staff member's actions, as their loved one did not want heroic efforts at the end of life, but a national conversation was started about the expectation of CPR in assisted living [31]. As with all other major assisted living policies, there is great variation state-to-state on the provision of CPR by staff. While current data are not readily available, in 2013 fewer than 20 states had regulatory requirements for assisted living staff to be trained in CPR. Some states, for example Colorado, mandated that a CPR-certified staff member is always onsite. Many other states did not have policies requiring CPR in the assisted living and allowed communities to determine if they will offer

CPR as an expected service or not [32]. Assisted living communities may have a "no-CPR policy" but are required to clearly inform residents and families of procedures to address emergencies and make it clear that in the event of cardiac arrest, staff will not start resuscitative efforts. Resident agreements should clarify that CPR will not be administered if a resident is found unresponsive by staff, so the policy is acknowledged before admission to the community.

Advance directive documentation, like Physician Orders for Life-Sustaining Treatment (POLST) and related forms are important aspects of a resident's care plan and should be completed with the medical provider and available to assisted living staff. Having active advance directives will help ensure that residents' wishes will be honored when they become severely ill or die. In the 2013 case in California referenced above, if the resident had an available POLST form, the question of CPR would not have come up and the controversy may have been avoided.

End-of-life care is often coordinated with hospice agencies, which bring specialized palliative services to the assisted living setting. However, the success of this model depends on the alignment between hospice capacity, assisted living staffing, and family expectations. For example, if a resident requires care that exceeds what the hospice and assisted living can jointly provide—such as continuous supervision for terminal agitation or specialized wound care—families may need to provide the care themselves or arrange for supplemental private duty caregivers. Effective coordination among the hospice team, medical provider, assisted living administrator, and the resident's family is critical for ensuring that end-of-life care is both feasible and aligned with the resident's preferences and the facility's licensure requirements.

Implications for "Assisted" and "Living"

Assisted living communities are now serving residents with increasingly complex medical, functional, and mental health needs, some of whom may resemble the population traditionally seen in nursing homes. Despite this shift, many communities lack the staffing, training, and infrastructure to adequately support higher-acuity residents, including those with dementia, chronic illnesses, and serious mental health conditions as evidenced by studies that show higher hospitalization rates for assisted living residents [33, 34]. A study in Oregon investigating direct staff to resident care time showed significant variability highlighting the great differences between communities in their structure and operations, staffing adequacy, and the heterogeneity in care needs among their residents [35].

A national survey of assisted living communities in 2022 determined that over half of assisted living communities were experiencing a decline in staffing rates with 63% reporting moderate or high staffing shortages [36]. In light of these issues, medical providers can serve an important role in ensuring their patients living in assisted living are truly getting "assisted" care. Medical outcomes are going to be more successful when medications are being administered as prescribed and patients have access to proper nutrition [37], both of which are mainstays of services provided in assisted living communities. With more direct coordination between medical providers and the assisted living staff, there will be fewer extraneous steps in care provision (fewer phone calls, faxes, and order clarifications) allowing the staff to be able to focus on the resident. Staff can often help optimize medical care by monitoring things like blood glucose and blood pressures under the orders of the medical provider, providing data and feedback to inform decision making. Coordination between staff and medical providers allows for residents to continue "living" in the community of their choice that provides social engagement and independence for as long as possible.

Assisted living residents are always walking the fine balance of needing just the right amount of assistance to stay in their community, and their medical providers are often tasked with making the determination of appropriate level of care. As the resident population grows more diverse and medically complex, regulations, financing models, and geriatric care practices must evolve to ensure both safety and resident autonomy are preserved.

Competing Interests The authors have no conflicts of interest to declare that are relevant to the content of this chapter.

References

1. AssistedLiving.org. AssistedLiving.org 2024 cost data methodology. 2024 Dec 15. https://www.assistedliving.org/cost-methodology. Accessed 14 Oct 2025.
2. American Health Care Association/National Center for Assisted Living (AHCA/NCAL). Facts & figures – assisted living. AHCA/NCAL. [cited 2025 Jul 2]. Available from: https://www.ahcancal.org/Assisted-Living/Facts-and-Figures/Pages/default.aspx.
3. Silver BC, Grabowski DC, Gozalo PL, Dosa D, Thomas KS. Increasing prevalence of assisted living as a substitute for private-pay long-term nursing care. Health Serv Res. 2018;53(6):4906–20.
4. Thomas KS, Belanger E, Zhang W. State variability in assisted living residents' end-of-life care trajectories. J Am Med Directors Assoc. 2019, Nov 6;21(3):415–9. https://doi.org/10.1016/j.jamda.2019.09.013.
5. Kelsey SG, Laditka SB, Laditka JN. Caregiver perspectives on transitions to assisted living and memory care. Am J Alzheimers Dis Other Demen. 2010 May;25(3):255–64. https://doi.org/10.1177/1533317509357737. Epub 2010 Feb 10.
6. Campbell-Enns HJ, Campbell M, Rieger KL, Thompson GN, Doupe MB. No other safe care option: nursing home admission as a last resort strategy. Gerontologist. 2020 Jun 26;60(8):1504–14.
7. Son JY, Marriott DJ, Struble LM, Chen W, Larson JL. Factors associated with transfer from assisted living facilities to a nursing home: National Health Aging Trends Study 2011–2019. J Am Geriatr Soc. 2024 Nov;72(11):3374–84.
8. Gaugler JE. Family involvement in residential long-term care: a synthesis and critical review. Aging Ment Health. 2005 Mar;9(2):105–18.
9. Resnick B, Allen J, McMahon E; American Assisted Living Nurses Association. The role of physicians practicing in assisted living: what changes do we really need? J Am Med Dir Assoc. 2018 Feb;19(2):104–5. https://doi.org/10.1016/j.jamda.2017.
10. Sloane P, Zimmerman S, Perez R, Reed D, Harris Wallace B, Khandelwal C, Beeber A, Mitchell C, Schumacher J. Physician perspectives on medical care delivery in assisted living. J Am Geriatr Soc. 2011;59(12):2326–31.

11. Sloane PD, Zimmerman S, Gruber-Baldini A, et al. Health and functional outcomes and health care utilization of persons with dementia: a comparison of assisted living and nursing homes. Gerontologist. 2005;45:124–32.
12. Dys S, Smith L, Tunalilar O, Carder P. Revisiting the role of physicians in assisted living and residential care settings. Gerontol Geriatr Med. 2020 Dec;10:6.
13. Nagurney JM, Fleischman W, Han L, Leo-Summers L, Allore HG, Gill TM. Emergency department visits without hospitalization are associated with functional decline in older persons. Ann Emerg Med. 2017 Apr;69(4):426–33.
14. Aminzadeh F, Dalziel WB. Older adults in the emergency department: a systematic review of patterns of use, adverse outcomes, and effectiveness of interventions. Ann Emerg Med. 2002 Mar;39(3):238–47.
15. Hua CL, Zhang W, Cornell PY, Rahman M, Dosa DM, Thomas KS. Characterizing emergency department use in assisted living. J Am Med Dir Assoc. 2021 Apr;22(4):913–7.
16. Roemer M. Costs of treat-and-release emergency department visits in the United States, 2021. HCUP Statistical Brief #311. Rockville (MD): Agency for Healthcare Research and Quality; 2024 Sep.
17. McGarry BE, Mao Y, Nelson DL, Temkin-Greener H. Hospital proximity and emergency department use among assisted living residents. J Am Med Dir Assoc. 2023 Sep;24(9):1349–55.
18. Mollot R, Whang S, Valanejad D. Assisted living: promising policies and practices for improving health, quality of life, and safety; 2018. https://nursinghome411.org/ltccc-report-assisted-living=promising-policies-and-practices. Accessed 22 Aug 2022.
19. Carder P, O'Keeffe J, O'Keeffe C. Compendium of residential care and assisted living regulations and policy: 2015. Addition. Available from: https://aspe.hhs.gov/basic-report/compendium-residential-care-and-assisted-living-regulations-and-policy-2015-edition.
20. Stearns SC, Park J, Zimmerman S, Gruber-Baldini AL, Konrad TR, Sloane PD. Determinants and effects of nurse staffing intensity and skill mix in residential care/assisted living settings. Gerontologist. 2007;47(5):662–71.
21. U.S. Department of Health and Human Services, Centers for Disease Control and Prevention, & National Center for Health Statistics. Residential care communities and their residents in 2010: A national portrait. 2016.
22. Temkin-Greener H, Mao Y, Ladwig S, Cai X, Zimmerman S, Li Y. Variability and potential determinants of assisted living state regulatory stringency. J Am Med Dir Assoc. 2021 Aug;22(8):1714-1719.e2.
23. Wang XJ, Teno JM, Rosendaal N, Smith L, Thomas KS, Dosa D, Gozalo PL, Carder P, Belanger E. State regulations and assisted living residents' potentially burdensome transitions at the end of life. J Palliat Med. 2023 Jun;26(6):757–67.
24. Caffrey C, Sengupta M. Variation in residential care community resident characteristics, by size of community: United States, 2016. NCHS data brief, no 299. Hyattsville, MD: National Center for Health Statistics. 2018 Feb.
25. Gillespie SM, Wasserman EB, Wood NE, Wang H, Dozier A, Nelson D, McConnochie KM, Shah MN. High-intensity telemedicine reduces emergency department use by older adults with dementia in senior living communities. J Am Med Dir Assoc. 2019 Aug;20(8):942–6.
26. Howd S. As assisted living evolves, medical directors can have a positive impact. Caring for the Ages. 2023 Nov–Dec;24(8):17.
27. Zimmerman S, Sloane PD, Wretman CJ, Cao K, Silbersack J, Carder P, Thomas KS, Allen J, Butrum K, Chicotel T, Giorgio P, Hernandez M, Kales H, Katz P, Klinger JH, Kunze M, Laxton C, McNealley V, Meeks S, O'Neil K, Pace D, Resnick B, Schwartz L, Seitz D, Smetanka L, Van Haitsma K. Recommendations for medical and mental health care in assisted living based on an expert Delphi consensus panel: a consensus statement. JAMA Netw Open. 2022 Sep 1;5(9):e2233872.
28. Zimmerman S, Sloane PD, Katz PR, Kunze M, O'Neil K, Resnick B. The need to include assisted living in responding to the COVID-19 pandemic. J Am Med Directors Assoc. 2020;21(5):572–5.

29. Post-Acute and Long-Term Care Medical Association. B09 – Physician's role in assisted living. PALTmed. 2009. https://paltmed.org/policies/b09-physicians-role-assisted-living.
30. PALTmed. Assisted Living Facility Medical Director Agreement. n.d. https://paltmed.org/products/assisted-living-facility-medical-director-agreement.
31. Berdzik CJ. Acuity level creep in assisted living. For the Defense. 2015 Aug: 48–51.
32. Are Assisted Living Facilities Required to Attempt CPR? [Internet]. Healthcare Law Insights; 2013 Oct [cited 2025 Jul 14]. Available from: https://www.healthcarelawinsights.com/2013/10/are-assisted-living-facilities-required-to-attempt-cpr/.
33. Hoben M, Hogan DB, Poss JW, Gruneir A, McGrail K, Griffith LE, Chamberlain SA, et al. Comparing quality of care outcomes between assisted living and nursing homes before and during the COVID-19 pandemic. J Am Geriatr Soc. 2023;71(10):3198–211.
34. Bartley MM, Quigg SM, Chandra A, Takahashi PY. Health outcomes from assisted living facilities: a cohort study of a primary care practice. J Am Med Dir Assoc. 2018 Mar;19(3):B26.
35. Dys S, Tunalilar O. Assisted living, residential care, and memory care staffing level dynamics: Oregon, 2017–2023. J Am Med Dir Assoc. 2025 Jan;26(1):105352.
36. American Health Care Association & National Center for Assisted Living. State of the assisted living industry: Survey of 120 assisted living providers show industry still facing major staffing and economic crisis. American Health Care Association & National Center for Assisted Living. 2022, June. https://www.ahcancal.org/News-and-Communications/Fact-Sheets/FactSheets/AL-Survey-June2022.pdf.
37. Fávaro-Moreira NC, Krausch-Hofmann S, Matthys C, Vereecken C, Vanhauwaert E, Declercq A, Bekkering GE, Duyck J. Risk factors for malnutrition in older adults: a systematic review of the literature based on longitudinal data. Adv Nutr. 2016 May 16;7(3):507–22.

Chapter 8
End-of-Life Care and Hospice

Emmanuelle Belanger

Introduction

Assisted living communities represent a unique long-term care setting, promising access to supportive care ("assisted") that has the potential to enable residents to live and age in place ("living"), in an enhanced, homelike setting. In practice, these communities provide residential care to a large population of frail older adults, many of whom require end-of-life care [1]. Even when they have worsening health and increased medical needs, residents often consider assisted living their home [2]. Yet, the regulations guiding residential care vary greatly across the US, and these communities are not all equally willing or able to manage complex medical conditions or terminal illness, especially compared to nursing homes [3]. With more individuals choosing assisted living [4], questions about the quality of end-of-life care delivered in this setting have become increasingly urgent. Research in this area has grown in recent years, but major gaps remain in understanding the interplay between state regulations, community organizational characteristics and care processes, and resident characteristics as they influence outcomes at the end of life.

This chapter reviews the current state of the science on end-of-life care in assisted living, with a particular focus on dying in place and the use of the Medicare Hospice Benefit. It begins with a national overview of the characteristics of assisted living residents who die in these settings and the common pathways of care they follow. Key factors associated with dying in place and receiving hospice care are then examined. The chapter concludes with practice recommendations and policy implications, as well as priority areas for future research if assisted living is to fulfill its promise of providing "assisted" and "living" care, allowing residents to live and age in place. To understand the role of hospice and end-of-life care in assisted living, it is essential to

E. Belanger (✉)
Center for Gerontology and Healthcare Research, Department of Health Services, Policy & Practice, Brown University School of Public Health, Providence, RI, USA
e-mail: emmanuelle_belanger@brown.edu

H. Temkin-Greener and S. Zimmerman (eds.), *Assisted Living Through Research, Policy, and Practice*, https://doi.org/10.1007/978-3-032-32088-9_8

begin with a profile of the population receiving these services and the broader policy environment that shapes the delivery of this care.

Characteristics of Dying Residents and Hospice Utilization in Assisted Living

This section explores the characteristics of dying assisted living residents and national patterns in healthcare utilization at the end of life. Assisted living is an important place of care for older adults with complex health needs, especially those with Alzheimer's disease and related dementia. National administrative claims data show an increase in the proportion of Medicare beneficiaries receiving hospice care in assisted living over time. By 2015, 18% of Medicare hospice beneficiaries dying in the community resided in assisted living [5]. Analysis of administrative claims from 2017 to 2019 indicates that 35% of a national cohort of assisted living residents died during this period. A majority of these decedents were 85 years or older (77%), and they had an average of six or more chronic conditions, while 70% were diagnosed with dementia [1]. These statistics paint a picture of a frail, vulnerable population, and show that end-of-life care is far from uncommon in assisted living.

The Medicare Hospice Benefit plays a critical role in supporting these residents. Given that licensing, staffing levels, and service provision vary widely in assisted living [3], hospice services often help fill important gaps. Under Medicare Part A, beneficiaries may elect hospice if a physician certifies they have a terminal illness (a life expectancy of six months or less), and if they choose palliative care over curative treatment and formally elect hospice coverage. Hospice services are typically delivered in the place a person calls home, including private residences, nursing homes, and increasingly, assisted living. Hospice agencies provide not only routine home care, but also continuous home care which is designed for patients in times of crisis, inpatient respite, as well as general inpatient care when symptoms cannot be managed in the home setting. Yet, the large proportion of assisted living residents who have Alzheimer's disease and related dementia creates challenges for organizing hospice and end-of-life care in this setting. The terminal decline that accompanies dementia is characterized by a prolonged period of severe disability, and estimating an accurate prognosis to determine eligibility for the hospice benefit remains a challenge [6]. In fact, the length of hospice stay is much longer in assisted living than in any other settings, raising questions about the appropriateness of referral patterns [7].

As mentioned above, electing hospice in assisted living has become widespread. Belanger, Teno, et al. [8] analyzed Traditional Medicare claims data from a national cohort of beneficiaries present in assisted living during their last month of life in 2018. Their findings showed that 56% received hospice in place, and 6% received the more intensive continuous home care level. The study used a cross-sectional design and focused on beneficiaries in large assisted living communities (with 25+ units), using a validated algorithm to identify residents [9]. Another cohort study, by Temkin-Greener et al. [10], included smaller assisted living communities and reported that 60% of residents died in place, and of those 84% were enrolled in hospice, underscoring hospice's central role in enabling residents to remain in assisted living until death. Complementing these national data, a state-level survey in Oregon offered a more localized picture. Bucy et al. [11] conducted a cross-sectional study using a stratified random sample of assisted living and residential care communities across Oregon. As expected, their results showed that hospice users were generally older and had significantly greater care needs than those not enrolled in hospice, including dependency in activities of daily living, need for overnight staff support, and two-person assistance with mobility.

Despite its importance, the quality of hospice care delivered in assisted living is not without concern. According to the Consumer Assessment of Healthcare Providers and Systems (CAHPS) Hospice Survey, next of kin of residents who died in assisted living report significantly worse care experiences than those whose loved ones died at home [12]. Areas of concern include poor communication, insufficient training for family caregivers, and difficulty managing symptoms such as pain and breathlessness [12]. These findings suggest that the setting in which hospice is delivered may influence perceived quality, possibly due to coordination challenges between hospice agencies and assisted living staff, or other issues with care provided in assisted living itself. Guo, Temkin-Greener, and McGarry [13] analyzed CAHPS quality ratings across hospice providers and found that those with a high volume of assisted living residents had significantly lower quality scores. This study used a retrospective design with national hospice claims linked to CAHPS data. Hospice providers with more assisted living patients scored worse in domains such as pain management, symptom response, and caregiver communication [13]. These findings suggest the need for better oversight and possibly tailored hospice delivery models in residential care settings, though later work by the same team offers potential avenues to improve quality [14]. Their analysis of hospice claims data from over 50,000 assisted living residents demonstrated a small but significant association between visits by both clinical and non-clinical hospice staff in the last three days of life and aggregated hospice quality ratings, particularly emotional support and willingness to recommend the hospice agency [14].

Hospice provides support for assisted living residents who wish to remain in place, minimizing distressing transitions and providing comfort-focused care. However, as explored next, many assisted living residents have delayed hospice referrals and experience transfers in their final days. These patterns raise important questions about the process of electing hospice in assisted living and how end-of-life care is organized.

End-of-Life Care Pathways and Transitions

State variation in end-of-life outcomes is striking among assisted living residents, making it difficult to provide meaningful national descriptions. For example, Thomas et al. [15], using Medicare data from 2016, found that the average number of days spent on hospice in assisted living in the last month of life ranged from 2.1 in North Dakota to 13.8 in Utah. This study linked decedent-level claims with ZIP code-level assisted living residence data, revealing not only wide disparities in hospice access but also potential inequities in policy execution and provider availability. Similarly, Belanger et al. [16], found that the proportion of assisted living residents dying in place varied from 18% in New York to 74% in Utah. The authors attributed these differences in part to state regulations explicitly allowing hospice or third-party care services to be delivered within assisted living, but also to other factors such as hospice market characteristics and geographic variation in aggressiveness of end-of-life care.

One of the key indicators of poor-quality end-of-life care is the occurrence of potentially burdensome transitions. Makaroun et al. [17], identified such transitions as hospitalizations or emergency department visits in the last three days of life, or repeated hospital transfers for conditions that could be managed in the community, such as urinary tract infections, pneumonia, or dehydration. Using bereaved family member reports from the National Health and Aging Trends Study, they found that such transitions were associated with lower ratings of end-of-life care quality and reduced satisfaction with communication and symptom management. Wang et al. [18], extended this work by analyzing 2018 Medicare data from a national cohort of 37,668 decedents who had been living in large, assisted living communities 120 days prior to death. The study used a retrospective cohort design and found that 19% of these residents experienced a potentially burdensome transition, such as hospitalization shortly before death. State-level variation ranged from 9% in Wyoming to 31% in North Dakota, again suggesting that regulatory and market-level factors may play a substantial role.

Despite hospice use being relatively high in assisted living, transitions between healthcare settings remain common. Belanger et al. [1] found that among a national cohort of Traditional Medicare beneficiaries residing in assisted living during the last month of life, 46% died in place without any transfers, while 13% had three or more transitions before death. Notably, over 20% of residents left assisted living before their final month, indicating potential gaps in capacity to support terminally ill residents or possible misalignment between family expectations and assisted living capabilities. Guo et al. [19] found that 35% of residents experienced any transition from assisted living in the last 30 days of life, and 17% were transferred in the final week. This study also used a national cohort design and stratified outcomes by state staffing and training regulations, allowing an exploratory look at how workforce requirements may mitigate transitions.

These patterns raise important questions about the capabilities and limitations of assisted living communities in supporting residents during the last weeks of life. Though some transitions may be appropriate or unavoidable, such as for falls or family preference, repeated, late-stage transfers often reflect insufficient preparation, lack of coordinated care, or systemic barriers to providing high quality of care on-site.

Determinants of Dying in Place and Hospice Enrollment

Better understanding of what drives end-of-life care outcomes in assisted living is critical for developing effective policies and care models. This section examines the associations between state regulations, facility and resident characteristics, and care outcomes such as dying in place and hospice use. Several studies have investigated these determinants using cross-sectional or cohort designs, primarily with national cohorts of Traditional Medicare beneficiaries, often linked to state regulatory databases or other sources of data about assisted living community-level characteristics.

In a 2022 national cohort study of Traditional Medicare decedents in assisted living during their last month of life, Belanger, Teno, et al. [8] found that 56% received hospice in place, and 6% received more intensive continuous home care. The study used retrospective administrative claims data for 2018 and linked them to detailed regulatory data on state-level assisted living policies. The sample included over 44,000 decedents residing in large AL communities (25+ beds). This study's key contribution was identifying the association between regulations and hospice utilization in assisted living, finding that residents in states with explicit regulatory permission for hospice use were significantly more likely to receive it (57.3% vs. 52.6%). The difference was primarily driven by greater access to continuous home care, suggesting that supportive regulatory language may improve not only access but also intensity of end-of-life services provided in residential care. Notably, the same study found that communities in states requiring any registered nurse staffing had a lower likelihood of using hospice continuous care (2% vs. 7%). This finding highlights the complementary role that hospice plays: in states where staff with clinical skills are mandated, assisted living staff may rely less on external hospice support for managing terminal symptoms. Conversely, in settings without such clinical infrastructure, hospice may be crucial in bridging those gaps, particularly as care needs escalate near the end of life.

Belanger et al. [16] also analyzed the association between state regulations allowing third-party services, such as home health or hospice, and the odds of residents dying in place. Their cross-sectional study linked 2018 Medicare claims to state regulatory data and found that supportive regulatory language was associated with significantly higher odds of dying in place, even after controlling for residents' clinical characteristics and hospice market factors. These findings underscore the relationship between regulatory oversight and end-of-life care trajectories.

However, the relationship between regulation and care quality is not uniformly consistent across studies. Temkin-Greener et al. [10], in a study published in Health Affairs, assessed the association between regulatory stringency and care outcomes. Regulatory stringency was measured by a complex composite score reflecting the specificity of regulations across staffing, care provision, and admission criteria. Their analysis of a national cohort study of assisted living decedents showed that higher regulatory stringency was associated with a reduced likelihood of experiencing any end-of-life transfers. Yet, Wang et al. [20], using a similar dataset and focusing on a more restrictive definition of "potentially burdensome transitions" (e.g., hospital transfers in the final three days of life), found no significant association between staffing or third-party service regulations and these undesirable outcomes. Guo et al. [19] added further nuance in their retrospective study using 2018–2019 Medicare claims linked to regulatory typologies. They found that states with more explicit requirements for staff type or quantity and for end-of-life training were associated with significantly fewer transitions. These findings point to the possibility that not just the presence of a regulation, but the level of specificity and operational clarity may matter for end-of-life outcomes. This body of research suggests that while some aspects of regulations may be protective, others may have less impact or may depend on how regulations are interpreted and implemented across states and types of licenses, an expected finding given the complexity of the licensing and regulatory landscape.

Assisted living community-level designations may also contribute to variation in outcomes. For instance, Wang et al. [21] examined whether assisted living communities with dementia-specific licensing or memory-care designation had better outcomes in terms of hospice utilization. Their 2024 study used a national cohort of assisted living decedents with Alzheimer's disease or related dementias and found that those in specialized memory-care settings were associated with significantly higher hospice enrollment rates. While causality could not be determined due to the study's observational design, the authors suggest that this specialization may either attract more medically complex residents or may be better equipped to recognize terminal decline and facilitate hospice referrals.

Resident characteristics are also influential; Temkin-Greener et al. [10] found that race and ethnicity were significant predictors of dying in place, with Black and Hispanic residents less likely to remain in assisted living through death. This may reflect disparities in access, cultural attitudes toward death and dying, and differential organizational processes across assisted living communities. The same study found that dual Medicare-Medicaid enrollment was a stronger predictor of dying in place, suggesting that financing plays a critical role in determining this outcome. These findings align with broader research showing that Medicaid beneficiaries are more likely to be transferred out of assisted living before death [22], and that racial and ethnic minorities continue to face structural barriers to hospice access [23]. Understanding these intersecting factors is essential for policy and practice recommendations, if we are to ensure high quality of end-of-life care for all in assisted living.

Practice Recommendations and Policy Implications

Experts in the field would readily call for more consumer education about variation in assisted living services and more standardized quality reporting [24]. However, meaningful improvements in end-of-life care arguably will require coordinated actions across multiple levels, including consumers, providers, policymakers, and researchers. For example, family members considering long-term care options should consider asking explicitly about admission and retention policies for dying residents with various health concerns and needs [2], as well as the community's history of collaboration with local hospice providers. While these conversations may be difficult, they are essential for aligning expectations and planning ahead. When selecting an assisted living community, families should also be aware of key community-level characteristics associated with better end-of-life outcomes. For instance, a few studies suggest that hospice utilization in place is significantly higher among residents of larger, for-profit assisted living communities [11, 25]. Larger communities may be more likely to employ administrative staff with the capacity to coordinate hospice services and to form stable partnerships with hospice providers because higher volume of beneficiaries makes developing these relationships more worthwhile. However, this should not be interpreted as a uniform recommendation given the variation that exists across different licenses and residential care settings; smaller or non-profit communities may offer highly personalized care, including a high commitment to retaining dying residents.

From a systems perspective, one major gap to provide evidence-based policy recommendations is the absence of standardized, publicly reported quality metrics in assisted living, especially as related to end-of-life care. While nursing homes have extensive reporting requirements through CMS's Nursing Home Compare and hospice providers report CAHPS scores, assisted living remains largely opaque. Developing and mandating metrics focused on hospice utilization, transitions in the last 30 days of life, family satisfaction, and resident retention during terminal decline would improve transparency and create incentives for quality improvement [12, 24]. States should also assess their own regulatory environments for alignment with best practices. As highlighted by Belanger, Teno, et al. [8], regulations that explicitly permit hospice care and allow third-party services are associated with higher rates of dying in place and hospice utilization. Comparing individual state regulations with top-performing states in terms of hospice utilization in place, such as Utah or Oregon [15], could also help identify areas for potential improvement. Importantly, regulations that contain vague or optional language may be insufficient to drive change.

Policies that support early integration of palliative care could also enhance resident outcomes in this setting as in many others. Although hospice provides important support, its use typically occurs late in the disease trajectory. Palliative care, in contrast, can begin much earlier and can help residents and families navigate complex decisions before crisis points occur. Pilot programs and grant-funded initiatives could incentivize palliative consultation services in this setting, especially in states with limited hospice penetration. Workforce training is another promising area of intervention. In a statewide analysis in Florida, Dobbs et al. [26] found that communities where more direct care workers had received end-of-life care training had significantly higher rates of hospice use. A subsequent randomized trial demonstrated the feasibility and preliminary effectiveness of a dementia-specific palliative care training in assisted living [27], with promising impacts on advance care planning documentation. These findings suggest that mandatory or incentivized training, particularly in dementia care and symptom management, could be a valuable addition to state licensing requirements.

Moreover, disparities in access to hospice and dying in place remain persistent across racial, ethnic, and socioeconomic groups in assisted living. These disparities are not fully explained by community characteristics and likely reflect a mix of systemic bias, communication barriers, financial limitations, and cultural preferences. Policymakers should support culturally tailored education and explore waivers and other payment models to ensure that dual eligible Medicaid and Medicare Advantage enrollees have equitable access to hospice and palliative care services [10, 22, 23]. Value-based payment models whenever assisted living communities have state Medicaid contracts could be another avenue to consider for policymakers, rewarding strong performance on end-of-life quality metrics, such as low transition rates, high hospice engagement, or resident and family satisfaction scores. Such models might also include bonuses for retaining residents through the end of life according to their wishes, avoiding transfers that are both costly and potentially distressing.

Finally, oversight of hospice agencies serving assisted living could be improved. Guo, Temkin-Greener, and McGarry [13] found that hospice agencies with a high share of assisted living beneficiaries often delivered lower-quality care. Regulators might consider targeting oversight and audits toward these providers or encouraging partnerships with agencies that specialize in complex symptom management and care coordination. Certificate of need (CON) laws, which require state approval before new hospice agencies can enter a market, could also play a role in curbing low-quality, for-profit growth and should be explored further [28].

Directions for Future Research

Despite recent advances, many unanswered questions remain about end-of-life care in assisted living. This final section identifies pressing research gaps and methodological challenges in studying end-of-life care in assisted living. Residential care represents an underexplored setting for the study of hospice and end-of-life care, with substantial uncertainty about the drivers of quality of care for dying residents. Research questions about end-of-life care processes and outcomes face the same challenges that plague other topics in assisted living research because of a lack of standard assessment data at the national level and extensive variation in state regulations, licensing, and required services. Though more stringent state regulations, and those explicitly allowing hospice, were associated with higher hospice use in assisted living in cross-sectional studies [8, 10], substantial regulatory changes would be needed to determine the impact of changing these regulations on residents' outcomes in states where these are not already enacted. There is also limited insight into why hospice providers with a higher volume of assisted living beneficiaries appear to have lower quality of care according to publicly reported quality ratings [13]. We must conduct additional research about the referral patterns from assisted living to hospice providers, and on potential interventions to improve quality of hospice services provided in assisted living communities. We need to know more about the referral process to hospice and how often this is driven by assisted living staff as opposed to outside providers.

Knowledge of national healthcare utilization patterns in assisted living has improved considerably with the use of Medicare administrative claims data to track beneficiaries across settings [9, 29]. This methodological approach enabled researchers to follow individuals over time, identify their location of care, and document transitions, including movement between assisted living, hospitals, skilled nursing facilities, and hospice. These datasets have become the foundation for many of the national studies reviewed in this chapter. Yet, we still know relatively little about the end-of-life care outcomes of assisted living residents who are enrolled in Medicare Advantage, which have now come to represent over 50% of the population [30]. Administrative claims data also lack insight into resident preferences; primary data or additional resident assessments would be necessary for a better understanding of how current care pathways align with these preferences.

Overall, there is a pressing need for additional data to determine whether community-level care processes, such as an organizational commitment to retaining dying residents [25], person-centered protocols guiding their care [31] or hospice attitudes of assisted living staff [32], may not be more important drivers of assisted living residents' outcomes at the end of life than the current patchwork of state regulations. Future research could help further differentiate between necessary and avoidable transfers, taking into account resident acuity, community resources and services across license types, and hospice networks. Meanwhile, policies and practice models that emphasize proactive care planning, staff training in dementia and end-of-life care, and hospice-residential care coordination are likely to reduce unwanted transitions and improve end-of-life experiences for residents and their families.

Implications for "Assisted" and "Living"

End-of-life care in assisted living communities is an increasingly central feature of long-term care in the United States. As the population ages, more older adults are choosing assisted living over nursing homes, often because it offers greater autonomy, a social environment, and a more homelike setting. Though additional research is needed about end-of-life care in this setting, strong partnership with hospice providers and improved staff training in end-of-life and palliative care have the potential to fulfill the original promise of "assisted" and "living." That promise would extend an array of supportive and palliative services to care for the residents through the end of life, assuring they live and age in place. Yet assisted living communities were not originally designed to deliver healthcare to dying residents, and many still lack the infrastructure, staffing, and training necessary to manage serious illnesses. As a result, assisted living occupies a complicated space at the intersection of social care and medical need. This chapter has highlighted both the promise and limitations of end-of-life care in assisted living. On a positive note, the Medicare Hospice Benefit provides a foundational layer of support, enabling a large proportion of residents to die in place with appropriate symptom management even in times of medical crises. States with supportive regulations and communities with strong hospice partnerships suggest that high-quality, resident-centered care is possible even in non-medical settings. Moreover, innovations in palliative care training and hospice care coordination offer a promising path forward for improving practice.

However, major challenges remain. Regulatory variation across states contributes to wide disparities in hospice enrollment and place of death. Many residents are still transferred out of assisted living in their final days, likely due to staffing limitations and other risk management concerns. Racial and socioeconomic inequities persist, and workforce shortages threaten the sustainability of assisted living care delivery more broadly. Much like in other settings across the US health system, improving outcomes for dying assisted living residents will require more than simple solutions. It calls for policymakers to align state regulations with the realities of aging and dying in place, for investments in staff training, relationship building with hospice and palliative care, and the cultivation of a culture that supports more open conversations about death and dying. Consumers would also need to be empowered with clear information about what different types of assisted living can and cannot offer at the end of life. Ultimately, the goal is not simply to reduce transitions between healthcare settings or increase hospice enrollment, but to honor residents' preferences and values, and support their families. Provided with enough resources, assisted living can offer a homelike setting for residents to live and die, and researchers have a lot to contribute to shape responsive policy toward providing them with person-centered care at the end of life.

Competing Interests The author has no conflicts of interest to declare that are relevant to the content of this chapter.

References

1. Belanger E, Rosendaal N, Wang XJ, et al. Characteristics and end-of-life care pathways of decedents from a national cohort of assisted living residents. Med Care. 2024;62(2):125–30.
2. Ball MM, Kemp CL, Hollingsworth C, et al. "This is our last stop": Negotiating end-of-life transitions in assisted living. J Aging Stud. 2014;30:1–13.
3. Smith L, Carder P, Hua C, et al. A national typology of health service regulation in assisted living. Gerontologist 2024;64(5); https://doi.org/10.1093/geront/gnad109.

4. Melekin A, Sengupta M, Caffrey C. Residential Care Community Resident Characteristics: United States, 2022. NCHS Data Brief, no 506; 2024. https://doi.org/10.15620/cdc/158327.
5. Teno JM, Gozalo P, Trivedi AN, et al. Site of death, place of care, and health care transitions among US Medicare beneficiaries, 2000–2015. JAMA. 2018;320(3):264–71.
6. Mitchell SL, Black BS, Ersek M, et al. Advanced dementia: state of the art and priorities for the next decade. Ann Intern Med. 2012;156(1 Pt 1):45–51.
7. MedPAC Report to Congress. Chapter 9: Hospice Services. 03-2024.
8. Belanger E, Teno JM, Wang XJ, et al. State regulations and hospice utilization in assisted living during the last month of life. J Am Med Dir Assoc. 2022;23(8):1383-1388.e1.
9. Thomas KS, Smith L, Gadkari G, et al. Identifying a national cohort of Medicare beneficiaries residing in assisted living Settings: an updated method. J Am Med Dir Assoc. 2023;24(10):1513-1517.e3.
10. Temkin-Greener H, Guo W, Hua Y, et al. End-of-life care in assisted living communities: race and ethnicity, dual enrollment status, and state regulations. Health Aff. 2022;41(5):654–62.
11. Bucy T, Carder P, Tunalilar O. Dying in place: factors associated with hospice use in assisted living and residential care communities in Oregon. J Aging Environ 2021;1–18.
12. Quigley DD, Parast L, Haas A, et al. Differences in caregiver reports of the quality of hospice care across settings. J Am Geriatr Soc. 2020;68(6):1218–25.
13. Guo W, Temkin-Greener H, McGarry BE. Hospice providers serving assisted living residents: Association of higher volume with lower quality. J Am Geriatr Soc. 2024;72(8):2483–90.
14. Guo W, Cai S, Li Y, et al. Hospice visits and perceived hospice quality among assisted living residents. J Am Geriatr Soc. 2025;73(7):2212–9.
15. Thomas KS, Belanger E, Zhang W, et al. State variability in assisted living residents' end-of-life care trajectories. J Am Med Dir Assoc. 2020;21(3):415–9.
16. Belanger E, Rosendaal N, Wang XJ, et al. Association between state regulations supportive of third-party services and likelihood of assisted living residents in the US dying in place. JAMA Health Forum. 2022;3(10):e223432.
17. Makaroun LK, Teno JM, Freedman VA, et al. Late transitions and bereaved family member perceptions of quality of end-of-life care. J Am Geriatr Soc. 2018;66(9):1730–6.
18. Wang XJ, Teno JM, Gozalo PL, et al. State variation in potentially burdensome transitions among assisted living residents at the end of life. JAMA Intern Med. 2022;182(2):229–31.
19. Guo W, Cai S, Caprio T, et al. End-of-life care transitions in assisted living: associations with state staffing and training regulations. J Am Med Dir Assoc. 2023. https://doi.org/10.1016/j.jamda.2023.02.002.
20. Wang XJ, Teno JM, Rosendaal N, et al. State regulations and assisted living residents' potentially burdensome transitions at the end of life. J Palliat Med. 2023;26(6):757–67.
21. Wang XJ, Cornell PY, Belanger E, et al. Do end-of-life outcomes differ by assisted living memory-care designation? J Am Geriatr Soc. 2024;72(8):2491–9.
22. Rosendaal N, Hayes SL, Wang XJ, et al. Likelihood of assisted living residents aging in place as a factor of dual Medicare-Medicaid eligibility at the end of life. J Am Geriatr Soc. 2023;71(10):3310–3.
23. Tobin J, Rogers A, Winterburn I, et al. Hospice care access inequalities: a systematic review and narrative synthesis. BMJ Support Palliat Care. 2022;12(2):142–51.
24. Zimmerman S, Carder P, Schwartz L, et al. The imperative to reimagine assisted living. J Am Med Dir Assoc. 2022;23(2):225–34.
25. Travis LJ, Thomas KS, Clark MA, et al. Organizational characteristics of assisted living communities with policies supportive of admitting and retaining residents in need of end-of-life care. Am J Hosp Palliat Care. 2021;38(8):947–53.
26. Dobbs D, Kaufman S, Meng H. The association between assisted living direct care worker end-of-life training and hospice use patterns. Gerontol Geriatr Med. 2018;4:2333721418765522.
27. Dobbs D, Yauk J, Vogel CE, et al. Feasibility of the palliative care education in assisted living intervention for dementia care providers: a cluster randomized trial. Gerontologist 2024;64(1):gnad018.

28. Gaines AG, Cagle JG. Associations between certificate of need policies and hospice quality outcomes. Am J Hosp Palliat Care. 2024;41(5):471–8.
29. Temkin-Greener H, Mao Y, Li Y, et al. Using Medicare enrollment data to identify beneficiaries in assisted living. J Am Med Dir Assoc. 2023;24(3):277–83.
30. Freed M, Biniek JF, Damico A, et al. Medicare Advantage in 2024: enrollment update and key trends. 2024. Available from: https://www.kff.org/medicare/issue-brief/medicare-advantage-in-2024-enrollment-update-and-key-trends/. Last accessed 5 June 2025
31. Schwartz ML, Lima JC, Clark MA, et al. End-of-life culture change practices in U.S. nursing homes in 2016/2017. J Pain Symptom Manage 2019;57(3):525–34.
32. Dobbs DJ, Hanson L, Zimmerman S, et al. Hospice attitudes among assisted living and nursing home administrators, and the long-term care hospice attitudes scale. J Palliat Med. 2006;9(6):1388–400.

Chapter 9
Quality of Life and Quality of Care in Assisted Living

Candace L. Kemp

Quality of life and quality of care are essential and consequential matters in assisted living. Yet, quality, as with the industry itself, is complicated and influenced by a host of factors, including struggles between the industry's past, present, and future, what it promises and realistically can deliver (and to whom), and the involvement of diverse, often conflicting values and interests [1]. In its original conception, assisted living emerged within the long-term care landscape as a social care model offering supportive services delivered in residential homelike settings in ways that uphold personal choice, dignity, autonomy, independence, and safety. This dual promise of "assisting" to meet individual's evolving support needs and promoting quality "living" while facilitating aging in place is highly desirable, albeit challenging to accomplish especially as the industry expands and evolves. As Zimmerman and colleagues observe, "Today's assisted living does provide assistance and enable aging in place with a good *quality of life*—but not for everyone" [2]. Understanding quality of life and quality of care, including how and why they vary, is at the heart of this matter. It is against this backdrop and the evolving assisted living context that this chapter provides an overview of empirical research on quality of life and care in assisted living communities while highlighting the social embeddedness and dynamism of these two broad concepts.

Understanding Quality

Understanding quality of life and quality of care requires a conceptual approach that attends to this complexity and dynamism. Originally conceived as an explanatory framework to conceptualize the intersection of formal and informal care, the Convoy

C. L. Kemp (✉)
The Gerontology Institute, Georgia State University, Atlanta, GA, USA
e-mail: ckemp@gsu.edu

H. Temkin-Greener and S. Zimmerman (eds.), *Assisted Living Through Research, Policy, and Practice*, https://doi.org/10.1007/978-3-032-32088-9_9

of Care Model [3] provides a holistic lens with which to understand quality of life and care and the ability to age in place in assisted living [4]. The model derives from a synthesis of theoretical and empirical work and reflects the complex, multifaceted and nuanced nature of daily life, long-term care delivery and support exchanges. Identifying the multiple levels of influence and how they operate is a critical step in understanding quality experiences, including successes, failures, and hence, potential quality improvement areas.

As shown in Fig. 9.1, assisted living residents are situated within care convoys (i.e., networks) comprised of an evolving collection of care partners, both formal/paid and informal/unpaid, who assist with activities of daily living and instrumental activities of daily living, socio-emotional support, and health care activities and coordination. Convoys can include residents' family members and friends, co-residents, staff, volunteers, external providers (e.g., home health, hospice workers). The composition and function of resident convoys, including their own participation in care activities and coordination [5], directly impact quality of life and care [6]. The interdependent and evolving nature of care needs and relationships means that the individual and shared experiences of residents and care partners shape one another, a fact that contributes to the complexity of quality and requires ongoing negotiation. Relationships are central to the delivery of person-centered services and care, however a relationship-centered approach to care broadens the scope to further emphasize interdependence, interactions, collaboration, reciprocal exchanges, and interpersonal connections among and between long-term care residents and their care convoy members [7].

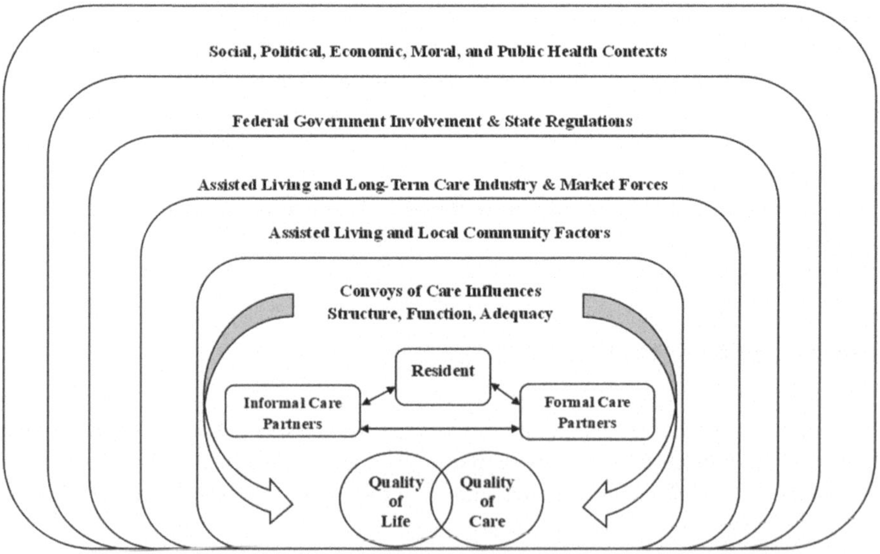

Fig. 9.1 Convoys of care and quality of life and quality of care in assisted living. Adapted from Kemp [3]

Multi-level Factors

Also shown in Fig. 9.1, the model adopts a socioecological approach and identifies the broader contexts within which care convoys operate and the myriad factors that intersect to shape quality at multiple levels. At the broadest levels, the social, demographic, political, economic, moral, and public health context along with federal and state regulatory contexts and industry-level factors exert considerable influence on assisted living. Unlike nursing homes, assisted living communities have historically been subject to relatively less regulatory oversight and quality assessment. In the absence of federal oversight within a largely for-profit industry, assisted living is somewhat of "a natural experiment" [2], that simultaneously generates opportunities for creativity and excellence as well as failures.

In 2001, the United State Congress held a hearing in response to the rapid expansion of assisted living and concerns over safety and quality. This hearing generated the landmark Assisted Living Workgroup Report (2003), which guided state-level regulatory expansion defining and re-classifying assisted living, establishing standards and reporting requirements aimed at quality improvement and encouraging transparency for consumers. State-level regulatory expansion further increased industry- and nationwide variability, especially in terms of regulatory requirements and stringency [8], care models and service delivery, payment models and access, and resident needs [1]. Consequently, Hawes and Phillips, in their seminal 2007 article, equate defining, measuring, and assuring quality in assisted living to "comparing apples, oranges, and broccoli" and describe these tasks as having "something of a Sisyphean cast" [9].

In more recent years, the industry has experienced additional rapid and fragmented growth fueled by an aging population, consumer demand, and profit margins with expanding private equity financing and involvement of the hospitality, real estate, and health care industries [1]. Paired with escalating levels of acuity and cognitive challenges among residents, these shifts further call into question the ability of assisted living, as an industry, to live up to the promise of providing care that meets resident needs, including the ability to age in place while promoting quality of life in a homelike environment [2]. Thus, despite being characterized as a social model of care, especially relative to the medical-institutional nursing home model against which it originated, assisted living can no longer deny the role it plays or needs to play in addressing residents' medical and psychosocial needs. This evolution has quality implications.

Coming under increasing scrutiny, assisted living has been at the focus of recent journalistic exposés and opinion pieces detailing neglect, abuse, preventable deaths, and lack of empathy, compassion, and respect for human life—the opposite of quality [10, 11]. The COVID-19 pandemic drew public attention to the essential and difficult nature of direct care work and the high turnover and low retention rates, which persist. Following the pandemic, the direct care workforce experienced even greater levels of burnout, anxiety, and depression, and reduced resilience [12]. Workforce issues, including who provides care and with what training, are consequential to quality in assisted living.

In 2024 and in response to mounting public concerns about safety, cost, and workforce issues, the Senate Special Committee on Aging, a body of the U.S. Senate that investigates and advises on issues affecting older American, convened a hearing to investigate assisted living and its care landscape, "Assisted Living Facilities: Understanding Long-Term Care Options for Older Adults" [13]. The concerns raised include the escalating cost and therefore accessibility of assisted living, resident safety and workforce-related issues and signal the federal government's continued interest in the industry.

These macro-level issues represent the broader framework within which individual assisted living communities operate. Individual communities themselves are, of course, exceedingly consequential in matters of quality and delivering needed support and promoting quality of life. As discussed later in the chapter, factors such as size, resources, location, connection to the surrounding community, hiring and training practices, staffing patterns and models, and resident characteristics, all shape resident experiences. Additionally, and returning to convoys of care, the characteristics of care networks and individuals, including residents (e.g., care needs, functional abilities, family involvement, care preferences, resources), family members (e.g., availability, involvement in care, nature of relationship), care workers (e.g., training, competence, confidence, care resources and behaviors), and others who comprise them, also are consequential to quality experiences. As alluded to throughout the chapter, individually and collectively, these multiple levels of influences intersect and have a bearing on who can live in and age-in-place assisted living, who works there, and with what implications for quality of life and care and individual experiences.

Defining Quality of Life and Care

Hawes and Phillps note that meaningful conceptualizations "of 'quality' in assisted living must embrace a variety of dimensions, including quality of care, quality of life, the physical environment, and resident rights" [9], all of which emphasize the resident experience. Qualitative research characterizes quality in assisted living as "a moving target" [14] that represents both processes and outcomes with overlapping domains that are structured and influenced by multiple factors at multiple levels all of which can change [4, 15]. Quality is highly subjective with definitions, standards, and priorities ranging, sometimes widely, among and between residents, family, staff, providers, and others [4, 14].

Far from universal, when asked about his definitions of quality of life and care, a resident's son said, "it's going to be different for everybody... In my mind, it's pretty simple. If I'm happy with it, [then] it's [good] quality," adding, "If Dad's happy, that's quality" [4]. Given the context-specific and multifaceted nature of quality, the overlap between quality of life and quality of care, and the diverse needs and preferences of the population and the range of perspectives and stakeholders [4, 14], it is neither likely—nor desirable—that a single, uniform approach to defining or assessing quality in assisted living will ever exist [16]. Nevertheless, along with finding ways to facilitate meaningful comparison, conceptualizing quality, identifying its various domains, and understanding the factors that lead to the most desirable outcomes, are essential activities.

Quality of life is a broad conceptualization that refers the assessor to consider the life of the assisted living resident more holistically and asks questions about whether residents are meaningfully engaged in life, whether they have autonomy, independence, dignity, well-being, and have a life that is directed by their own needs and preferences and that fulfills the human need to experience joy and the simple pleasures of their life embedded within a set of dynamic social relationships. The following explores a variety of quality-related topics that speak to the complexity of these two inter-related concepts. Generally, the usual conceptualization of quality of care refers to the specific evaluation or assessment of the care that residents receive. While the onsite care delivered by staff and a constellation of medical services typically though not always provided by outside parties [17], is almost always heavily supplemented by family and friend care partners [18], those who assess quality of care are usually focused on health care outcomes and the care received through these more formal and paid means.

Resident Well-Being

Beginning with well-being, several domains routinely appear in the literature and are understood to define residents' daily lives and lived experiences. Resident well-being is a foundational component of quality of life [4, 14], comprised of psychological/mental/emotional [15], physical, social, and spiritual health, all of which intersect with quality of care. Threats to well-being are often experienced during the initial move to assisted living [19, 20] as well as during times of crises or health decline, relocation within the community, particularly to a more advanced care unit, or other losses, including social relationships [21]. Well-being also can be compromised if there is overemphasis on one area of well-being to the neglect of others (e.g., prioritizing physical health over emotional well-being) [4].

Autonomy, Independence, and Choice

Autonomy, independence, and choice, principles of person-centered care, directly impact well-being and hence, quality of life [4]. Typically, and insofar as possible, most residents prefer to do as much for themselves and have as much control over their daily lives and care routines [5] including the ability to make or be involved in choices about where, how, with whom and when they spend time [4]. As residents experience declining function, care convoy members play increasingly important roles in supporting (and hence, also limiting) autonomy, independence, and choice in residents' lives. Many residents resent or resist restrictions on their ability to move about and do as they please, while some accept limits on autonomy, independence and choice as a trade-off for safety [14]. Often, residents adjust their expectations to match their ability to be autonomous, independent, and make choices and find greater satisfaction in smaller actions and choices [22]. Research on resident councils is limited but shows that these bodies can promote empowerment by including residents in decision-making and giving choice in decisions that affect their daily lives [23].

Physical Environment and Amenities

A care community's physical environment plays an essential role in quality of life and can promote or hinder resident well-being, independence and autonomy, engagement, and meaning-in-life [24]. Communities range dramatically in size, configuration, location, and ways that have implications for the social environment and safety. Locked doors and units are barriers but also can be critical to safety and can promote privacy. Private rooms contribute to feeling a homelike environment but may not be an option for many lower-income residents and those living in smaller, less resourced communities where non-kin room sharing is more common. The ability to personalize one's space, including having one's own possessions, also reinforces continuity, identity, personhood, and affects well-being [25], especially when transitioning to assisted living [19]. Such personalization can facilitate connection by providing points of reference for staff and fellow residents to gain familiarity, especially but not exclusively, for residents living with dementia.

A given community's configuration, design, and accessibility impact residents' autonomy, independence, and choice. Accessible wayfinding and environmental human-centered design features (e.g., lighting, flooring, carpets, signage, homelike design, safe outdoor spaces, accessible transportation) promote quality of life for a wide range of limitations including for those who have compromised vision or lower levels of physical or cognitive function. The availability of space both indoors and out that meet residents' preferences and needs is key to maintaining and improving well-being and quality of life [26].

Having accessible places of sufficient size and configuration to accommodate wheelchairs, walkers, and canes to facilitate safe navigation also supports quality of life. For many residents, having the ability to see and connect with the outside world, on- and off-site, including access to nature, is essential to quality of life, including for those living with dementia [27]. The amount and nature of a care community's amenities (e.g., activity areas, salons, courtyards, gardens, birdfeeders) and those in the surrounding neighborhood (e.g., sidewalks, crosswalks, parks, transportation), and their safety and upkeep, impact residents' well-being, social relationships, and engagement opportunities and experiences [27, 28].

Optimal Meaningful Engagement

Being optimally engaged in activities that are personally meaningful is a critical dimension of quality for assisted living residents [29], including those living with dementia [28]. Meaningful engagement can promote continuity, reinforce identity, autonomy and independence, social inclusion, and connectedness and is a fundamental component of holistic person-centered and relationship-centered care [28]. Engaging in activities that are personally meaningful also can promote a sense of purpose and reinforce the notion of meaning-in-life [24]. Engagement can maintain and improve physical and mental health [30] and represents a potentially effective non-pharmacological strategy to address several common conditions experienced by assisted living residents, including anxiety, depression, and behavioral expressions [31].

Engagement can involve physical, social, intellectual, artistic, and religious pursuits that take place individually, one-on-one or in a group with on- and off-site opportunities including those derived from self-directed activity, engagement programming and special events, daily life, and care routines (e.g., mealtimes, dressing), and presented by informal convoy members, especially family members [31]. Yet, not all communities have the same capacity to engage residents owing to variability in care partners' knowledge and engagement as well as community resources. In 2022, nationally, slightly more than half (55.5%) of assisted living communities employed an activities director [32].

Research shows that residents are often dissatisfied with activities and that engagement programming is consistently ranked as one of the weakest service areas [33]. Nevertheless, although participation frequency varies, the overwhelming majority of residents engage in some type of recreational activity [34]. Research also shows that residents in smaller communities are less likely to engage in leisure activities than those in medium and large communities and that those living in dementia-specific settings have higher activity participation rates relative to those who do not [34]. Activities are more apt to be passive than active [33], which has potential to negatively impact physical and cognitive health [35]. Staff availability and practices, residents' health, function, history, and preferences, as well as community layout, all can influence participation in physical activities [36].

Most residents (61%) go on outings although residents living in smaller communities and those with dementia are less likely to do so [34]. As with all residents, research by Ciofi and colleagues finds that outings among those living with dementia can provide meaningful engagement with nature, others, and the broader community [27]. Not all residents have opportunities to get out, typically owing to the absence of a facilitator. Getting out, while on balance positive, sometimes creates distress for residents or care partners, which underscores the importance of personally tailored engagement experiences, including possibly bringing the outside world in (e.g., through photos and movies, favorite foods or special events) [27].

Community activity programming frequently involves the creation of monthly or weekly activities to advertise offerings to residents, staff, and family members.

Research focused on residents living with dementia finds that care communities generally adhere to these calendars, yet activities are sometimes substituted with similar activities while others are canceled, which can leave residents with little or nothing to do leading to inactivity, boredom, disappointment and frustration, anxiety, and restlessness [37]. Factors influencing substitutions and cancellations included the availability of engagement staff, resources, and programming as well as limited direct care worker involvement.

Social Environment and Relationships

Living in a communal environment can guard against social isolation but does not necessarily protect against loneliness, which is commonly experienced among long-term care residents and has deleterious physical and mental health consequences [38]. This situation highlights the need to foster and prioritize meaningful social connection and honor residents' personal preferences for social integration. The social environment, comprised of relationships and interactions with co-residents, family and friends, staff and others within the community, and having the desired levels of social connection and intimacy including community integration are critical to resident quality of life [39, 40]. Positive social relationships are among the most consequential factors when it comes to feeling at home in assisted living [41].

Most residents have regular contact with family members [34], friends [42], and others, including former neighbors, co-workers, students, and church, sorority and fraternity members. Given the expectations of self-care and family involvement in assisted living, informal convoy members play pivotal roles that influence residents' quality of life through the provision of social and emotional support provided in person or virtually [6, 18], assistance with social integration and fostering positive relationships with co-residents and with staff [43]. Perhaps unsurprisingly, having a larger proportion of family members in one's social network is a significant predictor of resident well-being [42]. Yet, owing to competing responsibilities, residents' family members may have limited availability, and some residents have no family involvement or harmful family ties [6, 44].

Residents typically spend most of their time with other residents and staff, which makes these relationship partners extremely consequential to daily life [40, 45]. Co-resident relationships span a wide spectrum from strangers and neighbors to close friendships and even romantic partners [21, 40]. The nature of these relationships also varies widely with interactions ranging from supportive and friendly, to distant, strained, or in some cases hostile or abusive with related implications for quality of life [40]. Resident-staff relationships are similarly variable. Many relationships become close and family-like with blurred boundaries between formal and informal care [46] but others are less close, sometimes deliberately distant on the part of staff to avoid feelings of grief and loss that frequently are experienced when residents pass away [47]; still others are negative [3, 48].

Underscoring the importance of social integration, having some co-residents in one's social network and positive resident and staff relationships are associated with greater resident well-being [42] and quality of life [41]. Maintaining healthy levels of intimacy—broadly encompassing emotional, physical, intellectual, and spiritual connections, whether platonic or romantic or sexual—is a vital and frequently overlooked component of overall quality of life for assisted living residents [43]. Positive relationships in assisted living do occur naturally but typically benefit from deliberate cultivation. The overall social culture of a home is largely determined by its size, location, care model, resident and staff profiles, involvement of family, friends, and outside community members, as well as ownership, staffing patterns, care model, funding, and care philosophy and values. For instance, smaller and family-owned communities often provide more intimate social settings relative to large corporately owned communities that house more residents, employ a greater number of staff, and may be spread over multiple buildings [45].

Food and Mealtimes

Perhaps unsurprisingly, food and mealtimes contribute significantly to resident well-being [41] and quality of life in assisted living and are among the many sources of resident satisfaction and dissatisfaction [4, 24, 49]. Deeply personal, food preferences are rooted in life history, culture, religion, identity, and memories of home [14]. Meals, however, also need to meet nutritional standards and adhere to personalized dietary requirements/preferences to support health conditions such as hypertension, diabetes, or others. As such, they are a key feature of care delivery and quality. Food and dining experiences relate to and are influenced by resident needs, staffing configurations and availability of staff, cost, and related regulatory requirements [50].

Food aside, mealtimes structure daily life and provide consistent opportunities for meaningful engagement and social connection, representing "the center of everyday experience" [14]. Most residents look forward to meals, viewing them as a meaningful activity. The dining room is a social setting in which residents visit with one another and with staff during meal service, and can entertain their visitors, including family members, friends, and others. Even when there is limited or no mealtime conversations between residents, the dining room often is a site where co-resident support exchanges happen, especially among tablemates, by providing various types of assistance, including cuing, sharing, and ensuring others' dietary needs and preferences are considered [40]. The dining room also is a source of social divisions by making apparent differences in functional needs and limitations and the need for assistance which can result in "coming together and pulling apart" among residents [51]. Much like achieving optimal meaningful engagement for each resident, catering to collective and individual dietary needs and food and dining preferences is a complex challenge and an essential piece of the quality of life (and care) equation in assisted living. A recent systematic review of mealtime experiences in long-term care settings concluded that a resident's "capacity for agency to enact choices about menu, seating, social and environmental preferences, can be supported by policy, organizational and staff structures that respond to their needs and capabilities" [50].

Safety, Security, and a Sense of Home

Given the fact that most residents move to assisted living because they can no longer safely live alone or with others, residents, family members, providers, and staff all emphasize the importance of safety and security [4]. Safety encompasses elements of the physical design and environment, emergency preparedness with established protocols for fire, falls, medical emergencies, or natural disasters, which support physical safety as well as the social environment and social and psychological safety. Additionally, care-related safety relates, for example, to monitoring and oversight and the safe delivery of routine care, medication management, food preparation, and infection control.

Along with feeling safe and secure, the various subdomains of quality of life (and care) identified above, when collectively realized contribute to assisted living's promise of a homelike environment, which further enhances quality of life [39]. For some residents, assisted living becomes home but for others, home remains in the past and the setting is homelike or not at all like home. Among the significant barriers to creating a sense of home or homelike environments are tensions between quality of life and quality of care, especially when resident acuity levels increase to resemble those of nursing home residents [52].

Customer Service and Care Delivery

Residents are also customers and their relationships with staff and the care with which staff provide AL services, or "customer service" is an important dimension of quality. As a resident care coordinator shared, quality of care "is all about the residents, it is not about [any]body else in this building other than these residents. They are the most important, valuable piece of the puzzle." At the most basic level, delivering quality care demands meeting oversight, assistance with activities of daily living along with medication management and assistance, all delivered in timely effective ways that also adhere to resident preferences in all care domains. Typically, meeting care needs means providing assistance and care with empathy and responsiveness in collaboration with residents and convoy members [24]. As Anderson and Blair note, "what staff do and the way they do it has a very real and lasting impact on the quality of life of residents, and that impact lasts well beyond the interaction" [53].

The growing complexity of health care needs in assisted living, including care at the end-of-life, reflects the preference of the residents for a place where they can age in place and where services such as hospice, home health, and private care aides are provided when and as needed [54]. Without question, staffing is among the most consequential factors affecting quality of life and care [29] in assisted living in order to fulfill its premise of "assisted" and "living." The bulk of care is delivered by direct care workers or aides who make up 75% of the assisted living workforce; 12% are licensed practical or vocational nurses and 13%, registered nurses [55]. As with residents, most direct care workers are women. Yet, unlike those they care for, most are people of color, disproportionately immigrants, and economically marginalized with about half living under 200% of the poverty line and 22% receiving health insurance through Medicaid or another means-tested source [56]. These workers have among the most physically and emotionally demanding jobs and frequently heavy workloads.

Direct care work, as Scales & Lepore explain, "requires a mix of technical care-giving skills; health-related knowledge; infection prevention and control expertise; emotional intelligence and relationship skills; and problem-solving and decision-making abilities" [57]. Much is expected of this workforce, often with limited training, supervision, support, recognition, and limited to no opportunities for career advancement. Along with understaffing, high callout and turnover rates and the use of agency staff, these conditions interfere with care continuity and the delivery of person- and relationship-centered care, putting residents and staff at risk of harm. Developing, supporting, and uplifting this workforce are among the most critical pieces of quality enhancement.

Researchers have developed methodologies for identifying Medicare beneficiaries in assisted living that allow scholars to document assisted living population characteristics, especially pertaining to health care use and a variety of quality of outcomes [58, 59], including emergency department use, nursing home placement, and end-of-life care [60–63]. This method has been also used to examine assisted living residents' dying trajectories, revealing variability by state, dual eligibility status, place of death and hospice use [64]. Furthermore, highlighting the importance of staffing levels, analyses of Medicare claims data show that increased specificity in states' staffing regulations (e.g., identifying specific staffing levels or staff-resident ratios) is associated with reductions in hospital admissions among assisted living residents, including those living with dementia [65]. However, flexible or as needed, staffing regulations (i.e., requiring a "sufficient" number of staff rather than specific ratios) remain the most common model nationwide [66]; although recently Oregon began requiring the use of an acuity-based staffing tool [67], which serves as an important step toward more accurately meeting resident care needs.

Care Models and Quality Balance

Smith and colleagues' typology of state health service regulations in assisted living identifies distinct types of care models based on regulatory specificity as it relates to: medication management/administration, third-party care, skilled nursing, and licensed nursing staff [17]. The typology, which includes: (1) housing, (2) holistic, (3) hybrid, (4) hospitality, (5) health care, and (6) health support, serves as an important tool for research, policy makers, consumers, and advocates because it allows for meaningful comparisons within and across types. All six types were found across states with some states having multiple types. Learning how these types support or hinder quality of life and care, and for whom, would further enhance understanding of the "resident quality balance" (i.e., the resident/person and care setting/environment fit) [14]. In the assisted living context, "optimal fit" refers to a community's ability "to meet the competence and needs of residents, including autonomy, choice, health status, function, cognition, and social considerations" [68]. Given that residents and care settings are continuously changing, assessing this fit requires ongoing assessment to ensure there is proper balance between quality of life and care.

The contributions of family, broadly defined, and family involvement in residents' care are highly consequential factors in the balance equation. Along with social and emotional contributions, family members monitor, frequently oversee and coordinate resident care, provide ADL and IADL assistance, advocate and assist with decision-making, bring supplies, and can be invaluable partners in the delivery of person-centered care and care planning [3, 18]. Thus, they directly impact care. Care staff may feel supported when family members are involved and find it difficult to do their jobs when residents are without such support [18]. Residents' convoys of care vary by size, composition, and adequacy but operate best and support residents, family members, and staff when levels of consensus, communication, and collaboration are high within the network [6], on an ongoing basis and during crises [44, 54]. When convoy members work together (as opposed to apart or at odds), residents are more likely to age in place with good quality of care and life [6, 44, 54].

Negotiating Priorities and Navigating Tensions

Research by Burgess and colleagues shows that quality of life and quality of care involve a process of "negotiating priorities" or working out what is important for residents' quality of life and care at any given time [4]. The interconnectedness and dynamism of quality of life and care mean there are apt to be tensions between the two leading to quality imbalances defined by "quality dilemmas" and "quality conundrums." Quality dilemmas arise when there are differing quality of life and quality of care priorities between residents and their convoy members or within the convoys themselves. For example, although well intentioned, the COVID-19 pandemic and ensuing public health response prioritized infection control over social and mental health, especially for assisted living residents. The ban on visits from family members, friends, and others, along with social isolation mandates that relegated residents to isolate, caused considerable harm to residents as well as staff and family members [18].

A typical everyday dilemma involves conflict between resident preferences for autonomy and independence and care partners' preferences for safety. How dilemmas get worked out can be shaped by regulatory contexts, but they are largely negotiated and dependent upon communication and collaboration. Who exerts power (i.e., resident, staff, family members) and can make the final determination at any given moment is dynamic, which speaks to the importance of understanding all perspectives.

Quality conundrums, on the other hand, occur when resident care needs are so substantial that quality of life domains are largely overshadowed. In these instances, quality of life is defined almost exclusively by quality of care, in large part because care requires greater time and coordination and if left unattended may negatively impact quality of life, especially overall well-being. Thus, as one study concludes, "there is a hierarchy of quality" in assisted living such that "at the most basic level, quality of care must be met" [4]. Both quality dilemmas and quality conundrums are embedded in the murky moral landscape of everyday ethical decision-making in assisted living, and point to the need for ethically sound practices and a consideration of values and moral conflicts in advancing quality of life and care [48, 69].

Assessing Quality

Measurement of quality of life and care in assisted living has largely been conducted through scholarly research, within individual care communities or community chains with the capacity to self-assess, and as part of state regulatory oversight with emphasis on compliance and safety [70]. A wide range of methods, both qualitative and quantitative, have been used to study quality of life and care including in-depth interviews, participant observation, narrative inquiry, and quantitative approaches involving surveys and claims-based studies.

There is no shortage of tools with which to assess "quality" in assisted living, but not all are equally rigorous. Zimmerman et al. identified 254 tools, both measures and instruments, with the potential to improve quality [16]. This scan resulted in recommending 96 tools across five quality domains: (1) person-centered care, (2) medication management, (3) care coordination/transitions, (4) resident/patient outcomes, and (5) workforce, and also identified a significant gap in quality measures for staffing sufficiency. Researchers point to community variability in size and service provision as justification for recommending such a large number of tools noting, "the range of tools allows providers to identify those that are most relevant to their population, organizational characteristics, mission, and quality improvement goals" [16].

Shippee et al.'s recent (2025) scoping review of academic and gray literature on quality measurement in assisted living in the U.S. identified nine separate rank-ordered quality domains, each with multiple subdomains and accompanying indicators: (1) resident quality of life; (2) resident and family satisfaction; (3) safety; (4) resident health outcomes; (4) staff; (6) physical and social environment; (7) service availability; (8) core values and philosophy; and (9) care services and integration [29]. Additional expert panel discussions led to the identification of five overlapping themes: (1) quality of living experiences; (2) person-centered quality measurement; (3) broadening scope of assisted living; (4) experiences of people with cognitive impairment; and (5) diverse stakeholder engagement with an emphasis on the need to include residents' voices. This comprehensive work further advances efforts to make quality assessment routine practice in assisted living, demonstrating the overlap between quality of life and care as well as the range of viewpoints, perspectives, and indicators.

In a recent white paper, the National Center for Assisted Living highlighted the important role of data collection in quality improvement and encouraged the move from paper to electronic charting to facilitate data-driven care and comparison, and encouraged providers to engage in a national platform for doing so [71]. Most communities do not presently have the infrastructure or the necessary resources to make the move to electronic charting, data collection, and analyses. Moreover, successful implementation of these recommendations also is largely dependent on provider-driven evaluations and decisions about what to measure and what data to act on [72].

Quality in Assisted Living via Oversight, Regulatory Compliance, and Complaints Data

Licensed and regulated by states, assisted living communities are subject to oversight and enforcement of state and certain federal laws (e.g., Fair Housing Act, Americans with Disabilities Act). All states and the District of Columbia, Puerto Rico, and Guam, under the mandate of the Older Americans Act, operate Long-Term Care Ombudsman programs. These programs are directly involved in assuring quality by advocating, educating, supporting, responding, and working to resolve complaints and problems related to the health, safety, welfare, and rights of individuals living in long-term care settings, including in assisted living. State ombudsmen document and report their activities, including data on complaints, through the National Ombudsman Reporting System (NORS). Complaints can be initiated by a range of individuals, including residents, family members, staff, volunteers, ombudsmen, or others. Complaints are classified into twelve categories (abuse, gross neglect, exploitation; access to information; admission, transfer, discharge, eviction; autonomy, choice, rights; financial, property; care; activities/community integration and social services; dietary; environment; facility policies, procedures and practices; complaints about an outside agency; system/others (non-facility)), each accompanied by sets of subcategories.

Both aggregated NORS data, and data from individual states and regions, contain important metrics that could be, but are infrequently, used by researchers to identify weaknesses, understand and investigate complaint patterns, contextual research findings [37] and improve quality of life and care. Noting this "underutilization" Magruder and colleagues' analyzed complaints data from Dallas, Texas [73]. They found that relative to larger communities, residents from smaller communities had a higher ratio of complaints. However, complaint severity was greater in medium and large communities with proportionally greater complaints pertaining to "medications, falls, call lights, and staffing." There also were differences by community size in terms of who made reports. Residents in smaller communities were less likely to initiate or have family members involved in complaints.

Across the country, states monitor and conduct different types of evaluations to assess individual assisted living communities, frequently through unannounced inspections related to licensing or in response to complaints. In most, though not all states, the agencies overseeing assisted living also inspect communities based on complaint referrals from ombudsman [74]. States vary in how they oversee regulations with some states having limited human and financial resources to monitor and enforce regulations [74]. Nevertheless, data collected by state surveyors represent infrequently examined data sources for addressing quality.

What little research that exists demonstrates, as does the NORS data, the potential value of these data for understanding patterns of compliance and deficiencies. For instance, Tunalilar and colleagues' analysis of deficiencies data from Oregon found one or more deficiency in nearly 80% of licensing inspections conducted between 2008 and 2016 [75]. The top three deficiency citations were: (1) medications and treatments; (2) change in condition and monitoring; and (3) resident health services. When analyzed using structural and environmental data, the team identified certain structural (larger size, memory care designation, shorter administrative tenure, for-profit status) and environmental (rural location, lower unemployment, market concentration) characteristics associated with greater odds of having deficiencies. A community's likelihood of being cited and the number of citations decreased over time. Tunalilar and colleagues highlight the value of and need for ongoing analysis of these types of data, including consideration of the relationship between deficiencies and resident outcomes, especially those related to subjective experiences of quality and the delivery of person-centered care.

Roberts and colleagues' recent analysis of state websites found that all 50 states and the District of Columbia had assisted living websites [76]. Focused on quality, costs, and services information, their analysis found that nearly 69% of sites posted routine survey information, 43% posted complaints data with fewer posting information about life-safety surveys (16%), emergency planning (4%), and sprinklers (8%). They identify information gaps, especially pertaining to quality, and the need for greater website usability. How consumers use the information, what information they seek or need, and "whether and how providing... quality information affects … quality at the state level" remain unexamined and important future directions. Roberts and colleagues conclude, "*If services are not satisfactory, consumers can move. However, for the market to reward quality and for providers to feel pressure to improve services, consumers need reliable, accessible, appropriate, and usable information*" [76].

Quality Assessment, Satisfaction Surveys, and Report Cards

Regulations, as Zimmerman and colleagues note, "set the floor rather than the ceiling for expected care" [1]. Thus, citations, deficiencies, and complaints data demonstrate when quality is compromised but do not tell the entire picture, especially related to resident and family member satisfaction. Certain states including Minnesota, Oregon, Washington, and Ohio conduct and publish consumer satisfaction surveys. Minnesota's newly introduced Assisted Living Report Card, informed by work from Shippee and colleagues, combines findings from resident quality of life and family satisfaction surveys with state licensing and investigations reports on resident health, safety, and staffing [29]. Results are converted into a star-rating system that allows consumers to search by rank-ordering their preferred quality measure. In 2025, Minnesota's Department of Health and Human Services instituted a "peering" system based on care community size and location to create equitable and meaningful comparison [77]. Unsurprisingly, upon inspecting available information, resident quality of life and family satisfaction ratings do not always align with one another or with the licensing and inspection data.

Mao and colleagues examined Google online reviews of assisted living communities and compared these ratings with resident "home time," an outcome measured by the time spent outside of emergency rooms, hospitals, or in-patient hospice and other institutional settings [78]. Higher (better) Google reviews were associated with more home time, whereas assisted living residents in communities with no online ratings had lower home time. The authors conclude that consumers' online ratings may be useful in signaling assisted living quality. This approach, linking online consumer reviews with claims-based outcomes data represents a novel and promising avenue for examining quality.

Implications for "Assisted" and "Living"

Quality of life is a deeply relational and person-centered concept—expansive in scope and inherently subjective. To ensure that research meaningfully informs assisted living practices, it is essential to pursue conceptual clarity and prioritize the key dimensions of quality of life that matter most to residents. Similarly, the quality of care within assisted living is shaped by the foundational values, purpose, and scope of the assisted living model itself. Aligning research and practice requires not only conceptual precision on the scholarly side but also mission-driven clarity at the industry level. Central to this alignment is the need for rigorous attention to the ethical dimensions of everyday decision-making in assisted living communities.

As resident acuity levels increase, these challenges intensify, necessitating innovative models for collaboration, consensus-building, communication, and capacity-building across care convoys, within care communities, and the broader industry. Addressing these complexities also demands continued progress toward a holistic, consolidated, transparent, and publicly accessible framework for assessing quality, especially one that foregrounds both quality of life and quality of care. Such a framework would empower stakeholders, including residents, families, providers, policymakers, and researchers, to make informed decisions and cultivate high-quality environments that best meet individual needs.

Improving outcomes means embracing person- and relationship-centered care models that not only prioritize resident autonomy and preferences but also strengthen the direct care workforce through initiatives that enhance job quality. Educating family members about their roles in the care network and fostering collaborative relationships within convoys are equally vital. Building a shared understanding of quality, especially from the resident's perspective, will help care partners strike a meaningful balance between quality of life and quality of care and work collectively to honor resident goals and values.

Ultimately, quality of life and quality of care are inseparable goals and in the context of assisted living rely on the extent to which care convoys and hence communities successfully meet residents' dynamic support needs ("assisted") in ways that promote living well and aging in place ("living"). A focus on health care metrics and measurement is important especially among residents with the highest care needs and those with limited resources. It also remains critical not to lose sight of quality of life, including awareness of simple pleasures and finding ways to foster joy and living well even at end of life. While advances in regulation and person-centered practices have improved outcomes for many residents, wide variability persists across states, providers, and populations, including access to assisted living. Ensuring that assisted living fulfills its promise as a supportive, dignified, and health care setting requires continued investment in staff training and compensation, equitable access, data transparency, and strategic regulatory oversight. As the industry evolves, especially in response to meeting the needs of older adults with complex needs, the imperative is clear. Quality should be the lived experience of every resident and convoy member, especially residents' family members and friends and assisted living staff. Yet, myriad factors shape quality, many of which are competing, and lead back to Zimmerman and colleagues' conclusion that while assisted living is providing quality care and promoting quality of life, it does so for some though not all [2]. Understanding and addressing how and why this variability exists should continue to be a critical focus for researchers, professional organizations, practitioners, policymakers, regulators, and advocates, all of whom endeavor to improve assisted living experiences.

Ultimately, quality matters most directly to current and prospective residents, family members and friends, providers, and direct care workers and other staff as they are the ones who live, visit, and work in these settings or may do so in the future. Ideally, quality of life and care in assisted living also should matter to everyone else. Older adults and individuals who need support and the workers who provide the bulk of care in assisted living are members of vulnerable populations. Quality of life and care serve as indicators of the values, priorities, and individuals we, as a society, recognize and support [18, 79, 80].

Competing Interests The author has no conflicts of interest to declare that are relevant to the content of this chapter.

References

1. Zimmerman S, Carder P, Schwartz L, Silbersack J, Temkin-Greener H, Thomas KS, et al. The imperative to reimagine assisted living. J Am Med Dir Assoc. 2022;23(2):225–34. https://doi.org/10.1016/j.jamda.2021.12.004.
2. Zimmerman S, Stone RI, Carder P, Thomas K. Does assisted living provide assitance and promote living? Health Aff. 2024;43(5):674–81. https://doi.org/10.1377/hlthaff.2023.00972.
3. Kemp CL, Ball MM, Perkins MM. Convoys of care: theorizing intersections of formal and informal care. J Aging Stud. 2013;27:15–29. https://doi.org/10.1016/j.jaging.2012.10.002.
4. Burgess EO, Kemp CL, Bender AA. "It's going to be different for everyone": negotiating quality of life and care priorities within care convoys. J Aging Health. 2022;34(4–5):602–13. https://doi.org/10.1177/08982643211052367.
5. Morgan JC, Kemp CL, Barmon C, Fitzroy A, Ball MM. Limiting and promoting resident self-care in assisted living. J Gerontol: Series B. 2021;76(8):1664–72. https://doi.org/10.1093/geronb/gbab016.
6. Kemp CL, Ball MM, Morgan JC, Doyle PJ, Burgess EO, Perkins MM. Maneuvering together, apart, and at odds: residents' care convoys in assisted living. J Gerontol: Series B. 2018;73(4):e13–23. https://doi.org/10.1093/geronb/gbx184.
7. Gurung S, Chaudhury H. Relationship-centered care for older adults in long-term care homes: a scoping review. J Appl Gerontol. 2025;07334648241309761. https://doi.org/10.1177/07334648241309761. PubMed PMID: 39787049.
8. Temkin-Greener H, Mao Y, Ladwig S, Cai X, Zimmerman S, Li Y. Variability and potential determinants of assisted living state regulatory stringency. J Am Med Dir Assoc. 2021;22(8):1714-9.e2. https://doi.org/10.1016/j.jamda.2020.10.014.
9. Hawes C, Phillips CD. Defining quality in assisted living: comparing apples, oranges, and broccoli. Gerontologist. 2007;47(suppl 1):40–50. https://doi.org/10.1093/geront/47.Supplement_1.40.
10. Anand G. How not to grow old in America. New York Times. 2019 Sept 14.
11. Atlanta journal constitution. Unprotected: broken promises in Georgia's senior care industry 2019–2020. Available from: https://www.ajc.com/news/ga-senior-care-investigation/.
12. Novilla MLB, Moxley VBA, Hanson CL, Redelfs AH, Glenn J, Donoso Naranjo PG, et al. COVID-19 and psychosocial well-being: did COVID-19 worsen U.S. Frontline healthcare workers' burnout, anxiety, and depression? Int J Environ Res Public Health. 2023;20(5):4414. PubMed PMID: https://doi.org/10.3390/ijerph20054414.
13. Assisted Living Facilities: Understanding Long-Term Care Options for Older Adults: Hearing before the United States Sentate Special Committee on Aging (2024).
14. Morgan LA, Frankowski AC, Roth EG, Keimig L, Zimmerman S, Eckert JK. Quality assisted living: informing practice through research. New York: Springer; 2012.
15. Ball MM, Whittington FJ, Perkins MM, Patterson VL, Hollingsworth C, King SV, et al. Quality of life in assisted living facilities: viewpoints of residents. J Appl Gerontol. 2000;19(3):304–25. https://doi.org/10.1177/073346480001900304.
16. Zimmerman S, Cohen LW, Washington T, Ward K, Giorgio P. Evaluating measures and instruments for quality improvement in assisted living. Ann Long-Term Care. 2016;24(9):15–24.
17. Smith L, Carder P, Hua C, Zimmerman S, Sloane PD, Zhang W, et al. A national typology of health service regulation in assisted living. Gerontologist. 2024;64(5):gnad109. https://doi.org/10.1093/geront/gnad109.
18. Kemp CL. More Than A Visitor: families as "essential" care partners during COVID-19. Gerontologist. 2021;61(2):145–51. https://doi.org/10.1093/geront/gnaa161.
19. Mueller KE, Puymbroeck MV, Crowe BM, Davis NJ. Exploring constraints to well-being for older adults in transition into an assisted living home: a qualitative study. Can J Aging / La Revue Canadienne du Vieillissement. 2023;42(4):688–95. https://doi.org/10.1017/S0714980823000284.

20. Mueller KE, Marieke VP, Christy B, Crowe BM, Davis N. Measuring older adults' wellbeing when transitioning into assisted living facilities: a confirmatory factor analysis of the Mueller assessment of transition (MAT). Aging Mental Health. 2024;28(6):936–42. https://doi.org/10.1080/13607863.2023.2293054.
21. Kemp CL, Ball MM, Perkins MM. Couples' social careers in assisted living: reconciling individual and shared situations. Gerontologist. 2016;56(5):841–54. https://doi.org/10.1093/geront/gnv025.
22. Perkins MM, Ball MM, Whittington FJ, Hollingsworth C. Relational autonomy in assisted living: a focus on diverse care settings for older adults. J Aging Stud. 2012;26:214–25. https://doi.org/10.1016/j.jaging.2012.01.001.
23. Bonifas RP, Hedgpeth J, Kramer C. Evidence of empowerment in resident council groups: an examination of two leadership models in assisted living. J Gerontol Soc Work. 2013;56(4):281–98. https://doi.org/10.1080/01634372.2013.772082.
24. Mejia C, Severt D. Linking service quality attributes to meaning-in-life outcomes for residents who have transitioned to an assisted living community. J Gerontol Soc Work. 2021;64(2):151–74. https://doi.org/10.1080/01634372.2020.1830329.
25. Mansfield R, Burton AE. Exploring the meaning of quality of life for assisted living residents: a photo-elicitation study. Geriatr Nurs. 2020;41(6):812–21. https://doi.org/10.1016/j.gerinurse.2020.03.021.
26. Kawashima A, Jin X, Komatsu A, Niwa S, Shimada H, Arai H, et al. Individual- and facility-level factors related to quality-of-life transitions in older adults in residential facilities: a systematic review. J Am Med Dir Assoc. 2025;26(8):105721. https://doi.org/10.1016/j.jamda.2025.105721.
27. Ciofi JM, Kemp CL, Bender AA. Assisted living residents with dementia: being out in the world and negotiating connections. Gerontologist. 2022;62(2):200–11. https://doi.org/10.1093/geront/gnab113.
28. Kemp CL, Bender AA, Morgan JC, Burgess EO, Epps FR, Hill AM, et al. Understanding capacity and optimizing meaningful engagement among persons living with dementia. Dementia. 2023;22(4):854–74. https://doi.org/10.1177/14713012231162713.
29. Shippee TP, Akosionu-DeSouza O, Beebe TJ, Parikh RR, Brasure M. Measurement of quality in assisted living in the United States of America: a scoping review. J Am Med Dir Assoc. 2025;26(1):105355. https://doi.org/10.1016/j.jamda.2024.105355.
30. Theurer K, Mortenson WB, Stone R, Suto M, Timonen V, Rozanova J. The need for a social revolution in residential care. J Aging Stud. 2015;35(Supplement C):201–10. https://doi.org/10.1016/j.jaging.2015.08.011.
31. Mansbach WE, Mace RA, Clark KM, Firth IM. Meaningful activity for long-term care residents with dementia: a comparison of activities and raters. Gerontologist. 2017;57(3):461–8. https://doi.org/10.1093/geront/gnv694.
32. National Center for Health Statistics (NCfH). National post-acute and long-term care survey. In: Statistics NCfH, editor. 2022.
33. Plys E. Recreational activity in assisted living communities: a critical review and theoretical model. Gerontologist. 2019;59(3):e207–22. https://doi.org/10.1093/geront/gnx138.
34. Sengupta M, Zimmerman S, Harris-Kojetin L. Activity engagement in residential care settings: findings from the national survey of residential care facilities. J Hous Elder. 2019;33(2):120–39. https://doi.org/10.1080/02763893.2018.1534178.
35. Resnick B, Galik E, Boltz M, Vigne E, Holmes S, Fix S, et al. Physical activity and function in assisted living residents. West J Nurs Res. 2018;40(12):1734–48. Epub 20180321. https://doi.org/10.1177/0193945918764448. PubMed PMID: 29560808; PubMed Central PMCID: PMC6119542.
36. Bender AA, Halpin SN, Kemp CL, Perkins MM. Barriers and facilitators to exercise participation among frail older African American assisted living residents. J Appl Gerontol. 2021;40(3):268–77. https://doi.org/10.1177/0733464819893923. PubMed PMID: 31833788.
37. Sease J, Kemp CL. Examining engagement calendar deviations in assisted living: a focus on residents with dementia. J Appl Gerontol. 2025;07334648241306572. https://doi.org/10.1177/07334648241306572. PubMed PMID: 39686778.

38. Lapane KL, Lim E, McPhillips E, Barooah A, Yuan Y, Dube CE. Health effects of loneliness and social isolation in older adults living in congregate long term care settings: a systematic review of quantitative and qualitative evidence. Arch Gerontol Geriatr. 2022;102: 104728. https://doi.org/10.1016/j.archger.2022.104728.
39. Alomari E, Steinke C. Quality of life in assisted living facilities for seniors: a descriptive exploratory study. Nurs Open. 2024;11(3):e2084. https://doi.org/10.1002/nop2.2084.
40. Kemp CL, Ball MM, Hollingsworth C, Perkins MM. Strangers and friends: residents' social careers in assisted living. J Gerontol B Psychol Sci Soc Sci. 2012;67:491–502. https://doi.org/10.1093/geronb/gbs043.
41. Street D, Burge S, Quadagno J, Barrett A. Salience of social relationships for resident well-being in assisted living. J Gerontol B Psychol Sci Soc Sci. 2007;62B(2):S129–34.
42. Perkins MM, Ball MM, Kemp CL, Hollingsworth C. Social relationships and resident health in assisted living: an application of the Convoy Model. Gerontologist. 2013;53(3):495–507. https://doi.org/10.1093/geront/gns124.
43. Fitzroy AF, Kemp CL, Burgess EO. "I'm not terribly lonely": advancing the understanding of intimacy among older adults. J Aging Stud. 2022;61:101005. https://doi.org/10.1016/j.jaging.2022.101005.
44. Kemp CL, Ball MM, Jason K, Dillard Appel JA, Fitzroy AF. Communicative competence: responding to residents' health changes in assisted living. Gerontologist. 2020;60:754–64. https://doi.org/10.1093/geront/gnz119.
45. Kemp CL, Ball MM, Hollingsworth C, Lepore MJ. Connections with residents: "It's all about the residents for me." In: Ball MM, Perkins MM, Hollingsworth C, Kemp CL, editors. Frontline workers in assisted living. Baltimore, MD: Johns Hopkins University Press; 2010. p. 145–70.
46. Kemp CL, Ball MM, Perkins MM, Hollingsworth C, Lepore MJ. "I get along with most of them": Direct care workers' relationships with residents' families in assisted living. Gerontologist. 2009;49(2):224–35.
47. Bender AA, Kemp CL, Vandenberg AE, Burgess EO, Perkins MM. "You gotta have your cry": administrator and direct care worker experiences of death in assisted living. J Aging Stud. 2022;63: 101072. https://doi.org/10.1016/j.jaging.2022.101072.
48. Turner K, Kemp CL, Lesandrini J, Madison B, Donohue E. Bioethics in gerontology: developing a typology of ethical issues in assisted living. J Appl Gerontol. 2024;43(5):520–6. https://doi.org/10.1177/07334648231211471. PubMed PMID: 37982692.
49. Temkin-Greener H, Mao Y, McGarry B. Online customer reviews of assisted living communities: association with community, county, and state factors. J Am Med Dir Assoc. 2023;24(6):841-5.e3. https://doi.org/10.1016/j.jamda.2023.02.007.
50. Koh RTG, Thirumanickam A, Attrill S. How are the mealtime experiences of people in residential aged care facilities informed by policy and best practice guidelines? A scoping review. BMC Geriatr. 2022;22(1):737. Epub 20220909. https://doi.org/10.1186/s12877-022-03340-9. PubMed PMID: 36085034; PubMed Central PMCID: PMC9463738.
51. Sandhu N, Kemp CL, Ball MM, Burgess EO, Perkins MM. Coming together and pulling apart: exploring the influence of functional status on co-resident relationships in assisted living. J Aging Stud. 2013;27:317–29. https://doi.org/10.1016/j.jaging.2013.07.001.
52. Kistler CE, Zimmerman S, Ward KT, Reed D, Golin C, Lewis CL. Health of older adults in assisted living and implications for preventive care. Gerontologist. 2016;57(5):949–54. https://doi.org/10.1093/geront/gnw053.
53. Anderson K, Blair A. Why we need to care about the care: a longitudinal study linking the quality of residential dementia care to residents' quality of life. Arch Gerontol Geriatr. 2020;91. https://doi.org/10.1016/j.archger.2020.104226.
54. Kemp CL, Ball MM, Perkins MM. Individualization and the Health Care Mosaic in assisted living. Gerontologist. 2019;59(4):664–754. https://doi.org/10.1093/geront/gny065.
55. National Center for Assisted Living. Workforce 2024 [cited 2025 June]. Available from: https://www.ahcancal.org/Assisted-Living/Facts-and-Figures/Pages/default.aspx.
56. Kelly C, Morgan JC, Kemp CL, Deichert J. A profile of the assisted living direct care workforce in the United States. J Appl Gerontol. 2020;39(1):16–27. https://doi.org/10.1177/0733464818757000.

57. Scales K, Lepore MJ. Always essential: valuing direct care workers in long-term care. Public Policy & Aging Report. 2020. https://doi.org/10.1093/ppar/praa022.
58. Thomas KS, Dosa D, Gozalo PL, Grabowski DC, Nazareno J, Makineni R, et al. A methodology to identify a cohort of Medicare beneficiaries residing in large assisted living facilities using administrative data. Med Care. 2018;56(2):e10–5. https://doi.org/10.1097/MLR.0000000000000659.
59. Temkin-Greener H, Mao Y, Li Y, McGarry B. Using Medicare enrollment data to identify beneficiaries in assisted living. J Am Med Dir Assoc. 2023;24(3):277–83. Epub 20220220. https://doi.org/10.1016/j.jamda.2022.01.062. PubMed PMID: 35196482; PubMed Central PMCID: PMC9391528.
60. Temkin-Greener H, Mao Y, McGarry B, Zimmerman S, Li Y. Health care use and outcomes in assisted living communities: race, ethnicity, and dual eligibility. Med Care Res Rev. 2022;79(4):500–10. https://doi.org/10.1177/10775587211050189. PubMed PMID: 34623210.
61. Temkin-Greener H, Guo WH, Hua YC, Li Y, Caprio T, Schwartz L, et al. End-of-life care in assisted living communities: race and ethnicity, dual enrollment status, and state regulations. Health Aff. 2022;41(5):654–62. https://doi.org/10.1377/hlthaff.2021.01677.PubMed PMID:WOS:000796584600009.
62. Guo W, Cai S, Li Y, McGarry BE, Caprio TV, Temkin-Greener H. Hospice visits and perceived hospice quality among assisted living residents. J Am Geriatr Soc. 2025;73(7):2212–9. https://doi.org/10.1111/jgs.19532.
63. McGarry BE, Mao Y, Nelson DL, Temkin-Greener H. Hospital proximity and emergency department use among assisted living residents. J Am Med Dir Assoc. 2023;24(9):1349–55.e5. https://doi.org/10.1016/j.jamda.2023.05.002.
64. Thomas KS, Belanger E, Zhang W, Carder P. State variability in assisted living residents' end-of-life care trajectories. J Am Med Dir Assoc. 2020;21(3):415–9. https://doi.org/10.1016/j.jamda.2019.09.013.
65. Thomas KS, Cornell PY, Zhang W, Smith L, Hua C, Kaskie B, et al. The relationship between states' staffing regulations and hospitalizations of assisted living residents. Health Aff. 2021;40(9):1377–85. https://doi.org/10.1377/hlthaff.2021.00598. PubMed PMID: 34495716.
66. Carder P, O'Keeffe J, O'Keeffe C, White E, Wiener JM. State regulatory provisions for residential care settings: an overview of staffing requirements. Research Triangle Park, NC: 2016 Contract No.: No. OP-0030-1607.
67. Oregon Department of Human Services. Acuity-Based Staffing 2025. Available from: https://www.oregon.gov/odhs/licensing/community-based-care/pages/acuity-based-staffing.aspx.
68. Siegel EO, Bowers BJ, Carder P, Young HM. Assisted living: optimal person-environment fit. Res Gerontol Nurs. 2021;14(1):5–12. https://doi.org/10.3928/19404921-20201020-01. PubMed PMID: 2478777234.
69. Kemp CL, Lesandrini J, Craft Morgan J, Burgess EO. The ethics in long-term care model: everyday ethics and the unseen moral landscape of assisted living. J Appl Gerontol. 2021:07334648211049806. https://doi.org/10.1177/07334648211049806. PubMed PMID: 34647824.
70. Ramly E, Parks R, Fishler T, Ford JH, Zimmerman D, Nordman-Oliveira S. Implementing large-scale data-driven quality improvement in assisted living. J Am Med Dir Assoc. 2022;23(2):280–7. https://doi.org/10.1016/j.jamda.2021.12.025.
71. National Center for Assisted Living. WHITE PAPER: The Importance of Data in Assisted Living. 2025. https://www.ahcancal.org/Assisted-Living/Provider-Resources/Documents/NCAL%20WHITE%20PAPER_FINAL-1.pdf
72. O'Connor J. Data doesn't improve care. People do. McKnights Senior Living. 2025.
73. Magruder KJ, Fields NL, Xu L. Sizing up assisted living: an examination of long-term care ombudsman complaint data. Home Health Care Serv Q. 2018;37(3):158–76. https://doi.org/10.1080/01621424.2018.1474830.
74. Kaskie B, Xu LL, Taylor S, Zhang WH, Thomas K, Corenell P, et al. Promoting quality of life and safety in assisted living: a survey of state monitoring and enforcement agents. Med Care Res Rev. 2022;79(5):731–7. https://doi.org/10.1177/10775587211053410.

75. Tunalilar O, Lin S, Carder P. Survey deficiencies as quality indicators in Oregon assisted living communities. Gerontologist. 2022;62(8):1124–34. https://doi.org/10.1093/geront/gnab176.
76. Roberts M, Peterson LJ, Hyer K. The state of states' assisted living websites: Information available to consumers. Gerontologist. 2020;60(5):878–84. https://doi.org/10.1093/geront/gnz174.
77. Minnesota Department of Human Services. Assisted Living Report Card: Peering and Thresholds for the Resident Health, Safety, and Staffing Ratios. 2025. https://mn.gov/dhs/assets/MDH%20Survey%20Ratings%20Thresholds%20and%20Peering_accessible_tcm1053-692867.pdf.
78. Mao Y, Li Y, McGarry B, Wang J, Temkin-Greener H. Are online reviews of assisted living communities associated with patient-centered outcomes? J Am Geriatr Soc. 2023;71(5):1505–14. https://doi.org/10.1111/jgs.18192.
79. Armstrong P, Armstrong H, Daly T. The thin blue line: long-term care as an indicator of equity in welfare states. Can Woman Stud. 2012;29:49–60.
80. Armstrong P. Balancing the tension in long-term residential care. Ageing Int. 2018;43(1):74–90. https://doi.org/10.1007/s12126-017-9284-8. PubMed PMID: 128548508.

Chapter 10
Perspectives of Providers and Consumer Advocates Regarding "Assisted" and "Living"

Walter Moczygemba, Sheryl Zimmerman, Rita Altman, Jennifer Svoboda, and Elizabeth H. Wheatley

Introduction

While research is important to understand the extent to which assisted living accomplishes its dual mandate of "assistance" and "living," efforts to improve assisted living practices and policies must also be informed by the firsthand perspectives of those who operate these communities (providers) and receive their services (consumers and their advocates). Providers, a term inclusive of owner-operators, directors, and administrators, have on the ground experience; they are responsible for service provision and resident well-being and safety, maintaining regulatory compliance, and cultivating a stable and well-trained workforce, all while operating a financially sustainable business. These varied roles afford a unique perspective on the current and evolving nature of assisted living and the challenges and opportunities faced by

W. Moczygemba (✉) · S. Zimmerman
Center for Excellence in Assisted Living (CEAL@UNC), School of Social Work, and the Cecil G. Sheps Center for Health Services Research, University of North Carolina at Chapel Hill, Chapel Hill, NC, USA
e-mail: wmoczy@unc.edu

S. Zimmerman
e-mail: sheryl_zimmerman@unc.edu

R. Altman
Rita Altman Memory Care Consulting LLC, Mechanicsburg, PA, USA
e-mail: ritaaltman4@gmail.com

J. Svoboda
Sapphire Health Services, Portland, OR, USA
e-mail: jenn.svobo@gmail.com

E. H. Wheatley
Benchmark Senior Living, Waltham, MA, USA
e-mail: ewheatley@benchmarkquality.com

H. Temkin-Greener and S. Zimmerman (eds.), *Assisted Living Through Research, Policy, and Practice*, https://doi.org/10.1007/978-3-032-32088-9_10

the sector. Consumer advocates, as referred to in this chapter, include those with lived experience in assisted living communities—family members of residents and those whose responsibility it is to understand and respond to the challenges and opportunities faced by residents and their informal care partners. Consumer advocates provide support to residents, families, and other constituents, and have a unique perspective of how residents experience both "assistance" and "living."

Methods

To learn the perspectives of providers and consumer advocates as they relate to the key research themes explored in this book, two discussion groups were conducted in collaboration with the national Center for Excellence in Assisted Living at the University of North Carolina at Chapel Hill (CEAL@UNC) [1], the results of which are summarized in this chapter. Discussion group participants were invited by CEAL@UNC based on their expertise and experience in the field of assisted living. Eight assisted living operators, owners, administrators, and healthcare professionals representing communities diverse in size and geographic location participated in the "provider" discussion group. The "consumer advocate" group consisted of three individuals, including a family member of an assisted living resident and two members of resident advocacy organizations, one of whom has experience as an ombudsman. Frontline workers (e.g., nurses, direct care professionals, food service staff) who are essential to the resident experience were not directly included in these discussions; however, to better include their perspectives, a member of the consumer advocate group was a workforce expert. Many participants across both groups had extensive experience in dementia care, further enriching conversations regarding residents with complex care needs.

Each virtual discussion group was recorded and had the same format. Specifically, over the course of approximately one hour, participants were asked to describe what is working "especially well" and what is creating the "most challenges" in relation to each of this book's eight central topics; an additional "blue sky" question was asked, providing each participant the opportunity to describe ideal innovations and/or practices in assisted living from their perspective. A central theme from the discussion groups is that although this book and chapters are organized around eight distinct topics, the topics are deeply interconnected, with challenges and opportunities in one directly and indirectly impacting the others (see Fig. 1).

The narrative that follows was developed from each discussion group's responses. All quotations were drawn from audio recordings. Group members were provided the opportunity to comment on and co-author the chapter. Throughout the chapter, readers will encounter seemingly contradictory narratives—stories of challenges to deliver high-quality care in an industry striving to address residents' evolving needs, juxtaposed with examples of innovative strategies and a commitment to person-centered care and support. The experiences and perspectives shared in this chapter

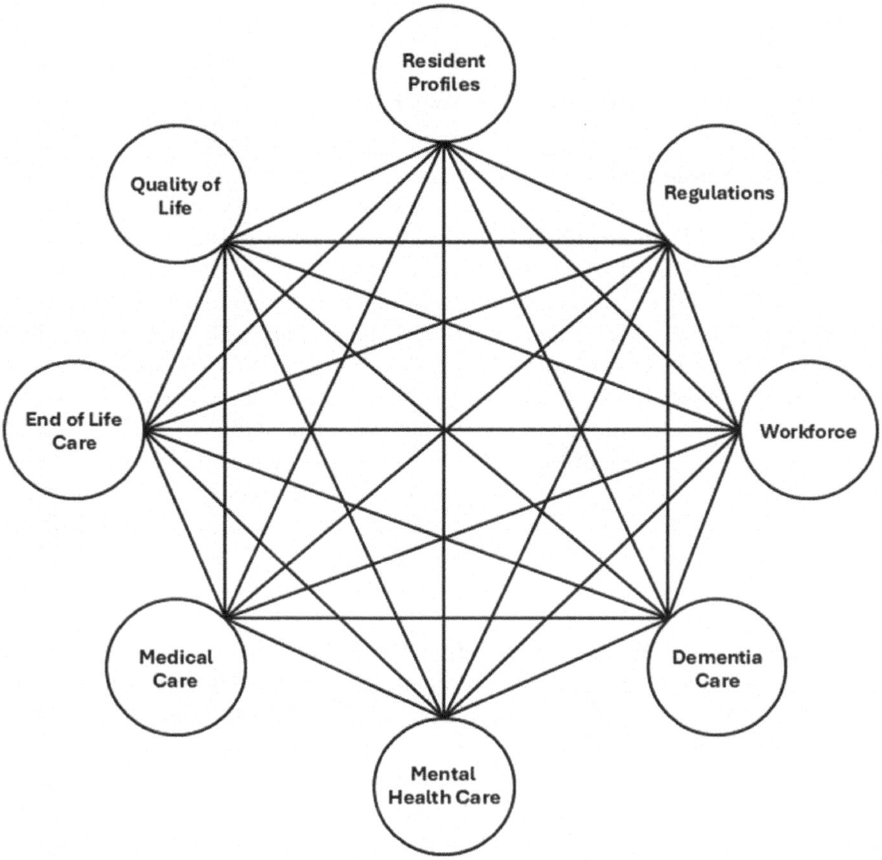

Fig. 1 The interconnectedness of assisted living challenges and opportunities

belong to those who provided them and offer insights into much of what is known, and what remains uncertain, about today's assisted living.

Authors' note: The perceptions shared in this chapter, while reflective of the discussions, do not represent those of all providers or consumer advocates. Toward that end, academic references are included to provide additional information and examples concerning specific topics.

Results

Who Comes to and Stays in Assisted Living

The Provider Perspective

Shifting Resident Demographics Providers described the assisted living landscape as continually evolving, driven in part by increasing life expectancies and a growing number of older adults desiring a social environment in which to live. They reported not only an increase in the number of current and potential residents, but also the complexity of their care needs. The rising number of residents with conditions requiring higher levels of care, alongside resource and regulatory constraints, presents difficulties for providers and challenges their ability to meet consumer expectations. Despite these difficulties, some providers viewed the changing demographic positively, noting that residents' evolving care needs provide the opportunity to broaden service provision; said one provider *"Who comes to assisted living is changing year by year. We're seeing people with more critical and diverse needs that we didn't see five or ten years ago. That's a good thing; it stretches us and forces us to enhance our capabilities"*

Successes and Challenges in Resident Retention Providers emphasized that assisted living offers more than just personal care, and that residents who actively engage in the social environment achieve a greater quality of life, saying *"[Residents] stay if they feel empowered, feel included, and if they still feel they have meaning and purpose in their lives."* Beyond fostering purpose through social connections, providers saw themselves as advocates to retain residents in assisted living, sharing information with residents and their support systems to help them navigate financial and logistical challenges to aging in place. One such example is providing information about the availability of resources such as Veterans Affairs Aid and Attendance benefits, which provide eligible Veterans with a monthly stipend that can pay for certain care services [2].

Affordability of assisted living was a pressing concern related to resident admission and retention; a provider described *"seeing an increasing number of people who have saved for retirement and want to be in a social environment, but they didn't save enough,"* an issue they emphasized will grow with time. For residents with moderate to complex medical care needs, providers estimated that assisted living costs easily reach $90,000 per year, and that even those who have purposefully saved for long-term care may find their funds insufficient, limiting their ability to age in place. Rising costs may necessitate creative solutions, such as private bridge loans or other short-term financial solutions to support residents financially while they wait for assets to come available, such as from home sale proceeds or insurance payoffs [3]. According to providers, rising costs stem in part from the need for more experienced and specialized staff including nurses who are paid at higher wages—which providers noted is influenced in part by an increasing number of regulations specifying nursing oversight and the growing presence of labor unions within the assisted living workforce—as well as by the limited availability of public funding.

Specifically, while public funding for assisted living is available in most states through Medicaid Home and Community Based Services (HCBS) waivers, many states have waiting lists due to there being a maximum number of individuals who may use the waivers at any one time [4]. Providers described the current state of public funding as having limited capacity to enable broad access to assisted living; indeed, in 2022 fewer than 20% of assisted living residents used Medicaid as a payer source [5].

During discussions on the challenges to affordability in assisted living, the existence of a feedback loop was mentioned, where the stress of navigating finances negatively affects residents' health status which can elevate their care needs and associated costs. Providers noted that these difficulties similarly impact residents' support systems, many of whom experience significant worry over how to fund care for their relatives.

Beyond financial concerns, providers described several other factors influencing resident retention, including changing care needs related to advanced age and multiple comorbidities and declining cognition due to dementia; some believed these changes play a more decisive role than finances in determining whether a resident can continue to age in place. Others noted that some residents leave simply because the communal environment does not align with their personal preferences or provide fulfillment.

The Consumer Advocate Perspective

Consumer Confusion Consumer advocates noted that consumers tend to embrace assisted living as their preferred long-term care option over nursing homes when an individual can no longer remain at home, even though *"many people don't know the difference between assisted living and nursing homes."* Consumer advocates suggested that this preference is in part driven by a negative reputation of nursing homes and the successful marketing campaigns of assisted living.

Consumer advocates highlighted that while assisted living communities market themselves as capable of accommodating a broad spectrum of care needs, their service limitations are not always clearly communicated, including related to staffing availability, service limitations, and move-out requirements. As a result, many residents enter assisted living assuming they can age in place regardless of their future care needs, believing that their current and future medical and mental health care needs can be accommodated. Indeed, for both consumers and providers, determining who is appropriate for assisted living is a challenge, and *"there is no hard and fast bright line in terms of who should be in assisted living and who should be in a nursing home."*

Further complicating the issue are differing state regulations and community-specific policies regarding the use of private care attendants and medical care in assisted living, with the variable accessibility of these options further blurring understanding of the distinction between assisted living and nursing homes. Echoing providers' descriptions of an evolving resident profile, one advocate described the profile of today's assisted living residents as similar to that of nursing home residents 20 years ago, with consumer advocates noting that in many cases it is quite difficult for families, individuals, and professionals to determine the most appropriate environment for a given prospective resident.

Decreasing Accessibility Consumer advocates, like providers, emphasized that affordability plays a crucial role in shaping who can enter and remain in assisted living, with assisted living increasingly becoming out of reach for most older adults. Consumer advocates described the lack of universal accessibility to assisted living as *"a huge area of concern when we think about it as a distinct model that is only available to a privileged few."* Because financial resources largely determine access to assisted living, opportunities for those who might benefit from living in a supportive care setting but lack the means to do so are limited.

The Regulatory Landscape

The Consumer Advocate Perspective

Room for Improvement Consumer advocates noted that current regulations have not kept pace with the evolving needs of assisted living residents. Unlike federally regulated nursing homes, assisted living is primarily governed at the state level, and consumer advocates described this framework as leading to inconsistencies in how assisted living is defined; workforce requirements; disclosure practices; resident protections; and mandated service limitations. They discussed that even states with rigorous standards may have notable gaps regarding the provision of medical care or accommodating varying care needs. Although consumer advocates appreciated the flexibility provided by state-based regulation, many called for enhanced standards to ensure consistent quality of care throughout the industry. One advocate explained:

> *"Increasingly, we are seeing state advocates pushing for higher levels of regulation to try and address some of the care concerns they are seeing. There is a lot of pushback from the industry which doesn't want to see assisted living [become] as highly regulated as nursing homes. I get it, but there has got to be balance in terms of ensuring that people's care needs are being met and their rights are being protected, yet still maintain flexibility and not have an overregulated system. That's been the biggest challenge: what is appropriate in assisted living?"*

Two areas with potential for regulatory reform identified by consumer advocates are resident discharge and resident rights. With the rising costs of assisted living and service limitations, advocates described situations wherein residents who are no longer able to fulfill their financial obligations, or who require care beyond the capabilities of their community, must move out, leaving them simultaneously lacking financial means and supportive care. For these residents, particularly those requiring specialized care, one advocate described the need for enhanced discharge protections to *"ensure that people are being sent to a place that can appropriately care for them, that there is a safe and orderly discharge,"* saying, *"these do not necessarily exist in assisted living except for in a few places."* In addition to discharges, consumer advocates noted that unlike nursing homes, for which federal Centers for Medicare & Medicaid Services (CMS) guidelines establish a clearly defined resident bill of rights [6], assisted living lacks a national framework, relying on varying state-mandated protections. Advocating for a national framework of resident rights, consumer advocates hoped to ensure uniform protections such as the ability to establish resident councils, a practice that they reported is expressly prohibited in some communities.

The Conundrum of Medicaid Consumer advocates focused on the particularly complex regulatory issues surrounding public funding for low-income assisted living residents. To use Medicaid funds for assisted living services, states must develop and maintain a Home and Community Based Services (HCBS) waiver program [7]. These programs, overseen by CMS, allow states to waive certain Medicaid program requirements in an effort to reduce the use of nursing homes for those needing long-term services and supports but not nursing care. However, consumer advocates described difficulties for both providers and consumers in understanding when certain federal CMS HCBS requirements apply to assisted living, saying, *"assisted living straddles that fence between nursing homes and true HCBS settings like independent apartments or home care; nobody quite knows what to do with assisted living."* Consumer advocates reported that in some cases, providers have ceased accepting public funding because of regulatory ambiguities and reimbursement limitations, further diminishing the financial accessibility of assisted living.

The Grey Market Consumer advocates described a growing segment of the assisted living industry that operates entirely outside traditional regulatory and licensure frameworks … *"an underground, unregulated, unlicensed, component of care… illegal, but not illegal enough to trigger a proper response."* The rise in these unlicensed communities [8], or "grey market," was attributed to a combination of factors such as the unaffordability of licensed assisted living communities, and members of the assisted living workforce feeling undervalued and underpaid, consequently deciding to operate directly from their own homes absent state oversight. Consumer advocates described these unregulated providers as catering to individuals desperate for supportive services but unable to afford or find licensed community care. While these services reflect a growing need for supportive residential services, consumer advocates expressed concern about this grey market due to the lack of visibility and regulatory accountability regarding care quality.

The Provider Perspective

The Effect of Regulation on Service Provision While state regulations for assisted living vary, providers noted that they significantly impact who can be admitted to, and remain in, assisted living. For example, states may prohibit assisted living communities from offering 24/7 skilled nursing care or require the discharge of residents whose behaviors pose safety risks [9]. Additionally, communities must navigate state-specific restrictions regarding the types of medical care needs that they can accommodate. These and other eligibility differences pose challenges for operators who manage communities across different states, and for families who live across state borders. One provider recalled the frustration of seeing families unable to access care in their own state due to restrictive regulations, while communities in a neighboring state with more regulatory flexibility could accommodate them. Still, providers widely valued state-based as opposed to federal regulation, seeing it as essential to maintaining the flexibility necessary to meet residents' diverse needs. When asked about the possibility of increased federal regulation of the industry, many providers felt that such oversight would impose rigid, one-size-fits-all standards, thereby limiting service models, driving up costs, and potentially decreasing quality of care. State regulation, they argued, allows communities to tailor services to their specific resident populations, preserving affordability and adaptability.

At the same time, providers expressed concern over inconsistencies in the way policies are enforced, particularly related to person-centered care. With high turnover among surveyors and newly hired surveyors often having limited operational experience, providers described inconsistent and impractical enforcement. As a result, regulations intended to support person-centered care were reported to be applied and enforced in ways that undermine its very tenets: *"from a regulatory standpoint, a lot of the regulations are written to be person-centered, yet in practice they are enforced in ways that contradict this approach."* One example provided was that of a former restaurateur living in a dementia care neighborhood who found meaning in assisting with dining services; the provider expressed concern that regulators might view the resident's involvement as unpaid labor.

Advocacy and Regulation Providers emphasized that robust advocacy is essential to develop regulations that are both realistic and supportive of the assisted living industry. For instance, one provider recounted a successful advocacy effort in their state; the proposed regulations would have required assisted living communities to provide dementia training to their staff administered by the state's Department of Health that was impractical to implement. By collaborating with legislators and the state chapter of the Alzheimer's Association, local providers developed a feasible training program that enhanced workforce education yet remained grounded in the realities of implementation.

Despite the absence of direct federal oversight, providers recognized the importance of advocacy at the national level. One example that was conveyed was the General Accounting Office calling for increased scrutiny of antipsychotic use for residents with dementia, about which a provider stated, *"there's a target on the back of assisted living providers."* Even if federal policies do not explicitly include assisted living, the ripple effects as described by providers—both positive and negative—can be significant. For example, providers voiced concerns over proposed federal mandates to increase staffing levels in skilled nursing facilities, fearing such directives would reduce the labor pool available to assisted living. To address these and similar challenges, providers advocated for coordinated, industry-wide efforts to increase policymakers' understanding of the complexities of assisted living and their role in long-term care services and supports. One area ripe for advocacy efforts involves the growing use of managed care plans for assisted living residents. These plans aim to reduce costs while also providing quality healthcare [10]. Providers expressed optimism that assisted living communities can demonstrate how their model effectively supports these dual goals and can be readily integrated into these plans.

The Role of Self-Regulation Some providers advocated for increased self-regulation within the industry. Suggested forms of self-regulation included using internal quality assurance measures or third-party credentialing bodies trusted to "validate" the delivery of high-quality care. Providers noted that adopting these voluntary community-specific approaches might be vital to the future of assisted living, complementing the accountability afforded by formal regulations, while striving to maintain high standards free from excessive regulatory burden.

> *"We do believe that companies and providers need to self-regulate…I think consumers deserve that. When done well, self-regulation can be a good guidepost to quality and service delivery that is person-centered and done in a way that is deserving of our constituent group."*

The Assisted Living Workforce

The Provider Perspective

Strategies to Expand and Retain the Workforce Providers agreed that the defining feature of an assisted living community is the staff, with a caring and compassionate workforce being *"more important than the building, more important than the programs, even more important than the food."* Given the importance of staff to the resident experience, it is no surprise that one of the most pressing challenges in assisted living is an ongoing workforce shortage. This shortage has led providers to make increasingly strategic decisions regarding resident admissions. When admitting new residents to memory care, for example, providers may become more selective as staffing constraints limit their ability to safely support residents and their dementia-specific care needs.

In response to these shortages, providers have implemented several innovations to expand the current workforce. Some communities collaborate with local nursing schools [11], integrating assisted living rotations into their curricula to enhance staffing while encouraging new graduates to consider careers in assisted living. Other providers emphasized the importance of broadening their recruitment efforts by "reimagining" what it means to be an assisted living caregiver, such as engaging retirees who may be interested in part-time caregiving roles.

Other strategies discussed by providers to strengthen the workforce focused on retention rather than recruitment. Some have introduced mentorship programs, self-scheduling options to provide staff with greater autonomy [12] and expanded compensation packages with childcare support [13] and same-day pay. Additionally, providers described embracing alternative career growth models, such as "career latticing," [14] a framework that encourages employees to grow not only through leadership roles but also by deepening their expertise in specialized areas such as dementia care or rehabilitation. By supporting lateral skill development, communities not only increase their overall capabilities but also retain experienced staff.

Technology as a Tool Amidst staffing shortages, providers are increasingly turning to technology to enhance efficiency and support their existing workforce. As stated by one provider, *"We're looking at how to leverage technology, not to increase staffing levels, but to allow our staff to be more involved in resident care… freeing up time so they can focus on resident engagement."* By streamlining operations through technology, providers can allow caregivers to dedicate more time to residents; automated tools can reduce tedious workloads, while mobile apps that integrate care schedules minimize the need for staff to return to central hubs to review care plans. Additionally, providers discussed the potential of emerging artificial intelligence (AI)-driven technologies, and the increased availability of data related to resident outcomes and health status to suggest care priorities and person-centered interventions based on documented behaviors.

The Consumer Advocate Perspective

Variability Among Staffing When asked to describe what is working especially well regarding the assisted living workforce, ten seconds of silence ensued among consumer advocates, with the conversation quickly moving to challenges. Consumer advocates described the same workforce shortages discussed by providers and observed significant variability among assisted living communities regarding staff preparedness and development. They reported that some providers who recognize the increasing dementia and medical care needs among residents are actively bolstering their nursing staff and enhancing training programs to meet evolving needs. In contrast, other communities remain static, with staffing numbers, skill sets, and overall staff knowledge not keeping up with residents' increasing care demands. Consumer advocates additionally questioned "*the extent to which those who are actually working in assisted living are even primed about the philosophical foundations of the model,*" namely providing person-centered care in a non-medicalized setting. Beyond increasing training, consumer advocates called for the restructuring of staff roles to foster increased empowerment and flexibility in care delivery. One such example was the creation of advanced frontline roles for unlicensed staff, including dementia specialist or peer mentor roles. One consumer advocate noted that these positions not only address community-specific needs but also provide much-needed career development opportunities.

Dementia Care in Assisted Living

The Consumer Advocate Perspective

The Growing Role of Dementia Care When discussing the successes of assisted living, one consumer advocate described, *"although with caveats, [the volume of] services for those living with dementia enables the opportunity [for persons living with dementia] … to live in a less medicalized setting."* With more and more older adults seeking support in a residential setting, the number of assisted living residents living with dementia has grown tremendously [15]. Consumer advocates discussed the benefit of a less clinical (i.e., non-nursing home), supportive environment for persons living with dementia, and noted that in many communities, individuals with cognitive impairment or dementia reside in the general resident population without receiving targeted, specialized care—and under the care of a workforce not always fully equipped to handle the behavioral, cognitive, and physical care needs that accompany dementia. Furthermore, due to the progressive nature of dementia, advocates noted that communities may eventually find themselves unable to continue providing adequate care beyond a certain level of need, resulting in state-mandated or internal policy-driven discharges, which are disruptive and emotionally difficult, especially for persons living with the later stages of dementia and their informal care partners.

The Uncertain Efficacy of Memory Care Memory care units, sometimes referred to as neighborhoods, have emerged as a prominent component of the assisted living model. However, consumer advocates reported significant variation in the success of these units, driven largely by differences in state regulations and operational practices. In some communities, they were thought to deliver high-quality, person-centered care, providing specialized services in a purposeful environment. Other communities were thought to fall short, with reports of residents being "parked" in front of televisions for much of the day, leading to a lack of socialization and engagement.

Consumers also questioned the utility of segregated memory care units, with *"units being hidden from view, both logistically and in more meaningful ways,"* resulting in a lack of data and public knowledge regarding the quality of care and quality of life afforded by these units. As an alternative, some advocates described care models wherein residents with dementia remain purposefully integrated in the broader community. Consumer advocates noted that if these communities maintain sufficient staff trained in dementia-sensitive care techniques, they may have the potential to better provide socialization and supportive services to residents who have cognitive impairment without segregating them from others.

The Provider Perspective

Preparing Staff to Provide High-Quality Dementia Care Providers uniformly stressed that effective dementia care depends on a well-trained, stable workforce; focused training is essential to ensure staff have the skills and confidence needed to provide high-quality dementia care. For example, providers described investing in virtual reality training programs that can simulate components of dementia such as confusion, disorientation, and frustration, creating a unique learning experience that can help direct care workers build empathy and understanding. These trainings may potentially serve a dual purpose, enhancing care by equipping staff with tools and techniques, and improving workforce retention by increasing the sense of competence and confidence in their roles [16]. Both are important to dementia care, and providers noted that frequent staff turnover severely limits their ability to develop the deep, individualized understanding of residents' history, preferences, and behaviors essential for person-centered dementia care.

Despite the wealth of tools and interventions designed to promote quality dementia care, providers cautioned that implementation is often inconsistent across communities. As one observed, *"I know we have an answer, but I don't know that it's always being executed."* Providers noted that strong leadership is needed to consistently promote and model best practices, lest even the best training programs fail to improve care quality. Additionally, the effectiveness of training relies on the quality of instruction and follow-through. To increase quality instruction, providers highlighted train-the-trainer programs that prepare experienced caregivers to effectively teach their colleagues, and implementing scorecard systems for trainers, describing these methods as "raising the bar" in terms of training standards.

Future Directions for Dementia Care Providers described a growing recognition of the risks of overreliance on pharmacological interventions to address behavioral expressions (e.g., resident agitation), noting that psychotropic medications have concerning side effects such as toxicity and increased falls. In response, some providers have focused on non-pharmacological approaches to dementia care, ranging from person-centered dementia care techniques (mirroring emotions, expressing empathy, validating feelings) to modifying the built environment. One provider reported that their organization has "*our own development company that's eager to hear about best practices to design buildings that can help promote independence and purposeful living.*" However, despite efforts to improve the built and care environment, providers noted that the assisted living industry is often "risk averse." Providers discussed worry about potential harm leading providers to place restrictions on residents' freedom and choice, resulting in efforts to honor residents' agency being a "tight rope to walk."

> *"With prospective residents often waiting until they are further in the disease process to move in, providers reported it a priority to expand service offerings to better accommodate individuals at different stages of cognitive decline. Describing a service gap between those with mild cognitive impairment and those with severe dementia, providers saw an opportunity for innovation within the senior living industry, stating, "another issue that is a challenge is*

having dementia-light versus dementia. I think we need to have a conversation [about that] in senior living."

Mental Health Care in Assisted Living

The Provider Perspective

A Lack of Service Providers From the provider standpoint, delivering effective mental health care in assisted living posed significant challenges. One described being *"hard pressed to find anything that's working well, to be honest; the challenge is finding resources, psychiatric physicians, nurse practitioners, and so on who are available to partner with us and have that same philosophy not to throw meds at everything."* Providers reported a widespread scarcity of specialized professionals within the workforce, namely a shortage of both geriatric psychiatrists and psychiatric or mental health nurse practitioners sub-specializing in geriatric mental health, thereby limiting their ability to provide specialized mental health services. Compounding this issue, providers described some practitioners as persistently using medications as the primary solution for mental health issues, running counter to more preferred, in assisted living, non-pharmacological approaches.

Evolving Needs, Evolving Care The challenges to providing mental health care in assisted living are unlikely to lessen, given growing and evolving mental health needs among current and future assisted living residents; the prevalence of serious mental illness in assisted living increased by over 50% from 2007 to 2017 [17]. Providers described shifting societal views of mental health that increase the demand for services in their communities, accompanied by an increasing acceptance of counseling among the baby boomer generation and their children. To meet these needs, communities are increasingly integrating telehealth services into their practices to expand their capacity. However, providers cautioned that telehealth may sometimes lead to an overreliance on medications and may require on-site nursing to facilitate visits.

In addition to telehealth, a few communities have begun offering programs for residents to undergo genetic testing to provide prescribers information on how their unique body chemistry will respond to specific antidepressants or other mental health medications, a novel approach that while promising, depends on private pay. Another provider looked further to the future: *"I'm somewhat intrigued about the future, but I worry too, coming right behind there's more PTSD. [And] for the folks on the autism spectrum, what will their needs be? What does that look like for assisted living? I'm not sure yet, but we need to be talking about this now as an industry".*

The Consumer Advocate Perspective

A Lack of Services Consumer advocates observed that while mental and behavioral healthcare is often incorporated into memory care for residents with dementia, serious questions remain about whether the current model of assisted living adequately addresses residents' broader mental health needs. In particular, consumer advocates highlighted a significant gap in staff training and expertise; one noted that *"we don't hear from staff that they're trained properly to handle the types of issues that arise; they don't know how to care for them [residents experiencing dementia- and mental health-related behavioral expressions], and that leaves both the staff and the residents vulnerable."* While the underlying reasons behind the seeming lack of attention to mental health in assisted living are complex, one potential explanation offered by consumer advocates is that individuals with related behavioral expressions may be more likely to be dually eligible for Medicaid, and may therefore more often reside in skilled nursing facilities than assisted living communities, causing a greater focus on mental health needs and training in those settings compared to assisted living.

Medical Care

The Consumer Advocate Perspective

Ambiguity and Appropriateness As previously described, the increasing acuity of assisted living residents as well as variations in state regulations may contribute to some confusion as to what services can and cannot be provided in assisted living. Consumer advocates noted that such ambiguity often starts well before a resident enters the community, given that even physicians—whose recommendations they described as often determining suitability for assisted living—are often not fully informed about the differences between assisted living and nursing home care. One advocate explained, *"Physicians are more clueless than we are in terms of who goes where, and what issues are involved in making that decision."*

The lack of clarity regarding which medical conditions may or may not be appropriate for assisted living extends beyond initial placement. Advocates noted that many who work in assisted living remain uncertain about the scope of medical care they can offer; one stated, *"Even within the assisted living community, those who are responsible for managing and providing services don't necessarily know what they are able to provide or not provide, or allowed to provide, or not provide."* Another recounted their experience helping their father, a resident in an assisted living community, navigate his temporarily increased medical care needs following surgery, specifically care related to a vacuum assisted closure of a wound. The process was described as *"the most incredible, tortuous set of conversations,"* during which their family encountered conflicting answers from different staff members and administrators regarding what the community could accommodate.

The Provider Perspective

The Role of Interdisciplinary Care Providers expressed optimism regarding their capacity to provide holistic, person-centered, medical care for residents. To do so, they described the importance of interdisciplinary teams as *"none of us can do this work alone; it takes an interdisciplinary, interprofessional team. The lone rangers out there trying to manage that care by themselves, that is totally inappropriate."* At the same time, varying professional involvement and models of care must be coordinated by a team leader, or "quarterback." Providers noted that while this role traditionally belongs to the primary care physician, in many assisted living communities, a director of nursing (DON) may fulfill this responsibility. However, there is no universal requirement for a DON in this care setting, with regulations varying by state and license type.

When discussing interdisciplinary care, providers identified two specific models as exemplifying the collaborative approach from which assisted living communities could potentially benefit: Institutional-Equivalent Special Needs Plans (IE-SNP) and the Guiding an Improved Dementia Experience (GUIDE) model.IE-SNPs, a facet of Medicare Advantage plans, can provide coverage for varying care needs by assigning dedicated care team members, such as a nurse practitioner and/or registered nurse, to serve as an on-site coordinator of care. These providers work closely with the resident's primary care physician, community staff, and other professionals, with the goal of providing residents with care tailored to their individual needs [18]. During group discussions, one provider commented about involving as many of their residents as possible in these plans after witnessing resulting reductions in hospitalization rates and decreasing instances of polypharmacy. The GUIDE model, operated by CMS, takes a specialized approach to interdisciplinary medical care for persons living with dementia and their care partners. This integrated care model prioritizes the individual's goals and uses alternative Medicare payment methods to assign a care navigator to individuals with dementia. The navigator's role is to facilitate access to essential medical and non-healthcare-related services and support while also providing caregiver support [19]. Despite being relatively new, providers expressed excitement about the potential for this and other forms of value-based care to be integrated into assisted living.

End-of-Life Care and Hospice

The Provider Perspective

Support in End-of-Life Care When describing the provision of end-of-life care in assisted living, one provider recalled seeing *"beautiful end-of-life journeys happen in assisted living"* enabled by several factors. Providers noted that state regulations may allow for additional services and greater care flexibility at the end of life, and that assisted living communities have become increasingly adept at coordinating with hospice and palliative care providers. Providers described taking a proactive approach to end-of-life care, initiating conversations early in the dying process, and educating residents and families on the differences between palliative and hospice care. Providers emphasized the importance of maintaining relationships with trusted external hospice and palliative care agencies that have delivered positive experiences. On the other hand, they also described having to function as resident advocates when external end-of-life care proved suboptimal.

Providers recognized the emotional toll that dying "in place" can take on those who provide care: "*I've seen really beautiful interactions and connections between a resident who is passing and an associate and the family involved in that, and I always have this guilt that we just don't do enough to truly appreciate the impact that it has on our teams when someone dies in our community.*" They noted that while some organizations coordinate with hospice and other agencies to offer bereavement support to their care staff, others fail to attend to the impact of working alongside death and dying for their staff, risking caregiver burnout and potentially exacerbating workforce shortages.

Limitations of End-of-Life Care Despite providers' optimism about the ability of assisted living to support end-of-life care, limitations remain. Some described pain management, often a priority during end-of-life care, as sometimes challenged by state regulations. Additionally, community-level resource limitations can hinder the delivery of continuous, 24/7 one-on-one care that may be necessary during the end of life. One provider explained,

> *"The challenge comes in when we may not have the staffing to come in and assist with helping them eat every meal, and the family may not be able to...and hospice doesn't provide that service...it's when there's particular services that the resident or family isn't able to pay for. Unfortunately, the conversations need to change."*

The Consumer Advocate Perspective

Ethical Concerns and End-of-Life Care Although discussions about end-of-life care among consumer advocates were brief, two key issues emerged. They questioned the extent of resident choice in selecting hospice care providers, noting a general lack of clarity about available options, and wondered how often it is that "*your only provider options are people that the assisted living facility contracts with?*" Another significant concern related to the shortage of licensed medical and nursing staff within communities. Given assisted living's focus on maintaining a non-medicalized environment, and general workforce shortages, many communities have limited nursing or medical expertise on staff. One consumer advocate illustrated the consequences of this as related to end of life:

> *"A colleague's mother is living in assisted living and has a DNR [do not resuscitate] order. The assisted living provider told her that their policy is that everyone gets CPR [cardiopulmonary resuscitation], it doesn't matter if they have a DNR order. Their policy is to provide CPR to everyone and call an ambulance, and when the ambulance comes, they are the ones who determine whether they are going to continue...this [act of disregarding a DNR] is a rights violation."*

Consumer advocates explained that while such practices are not universal, they are not unheard of, and attributed the situation to a combination of regulatory guidelines and the absence of licensed professionals capable of accurately assessing and managing medical emergencies in assisted living.

Quality of Care and Quality of Life

The Consumer Advocate Perspective

Variability of Care Consumer advocates highlighted significant differences in both the quality of care and quality of life between and within assisted living communities. They pointed out that within the same community, residents with light care needs, robust support networks, and retained capabilities often enjoy a higher quality of life and care compared to those whose care needs increase when external support does not. When describing variations between small-scale communities in their home-state, one advocate noted, *"It's like the tale of two cities. It's the best of care, it's the worst of care; a good small homelike facility can be terrific, just terrific; it can also be just terrible."* While consumer advocates noted that such variations stem from multiple factors, including financial resources, varying state regulations, and administrative structure, they consistently emphasized the important role of staff training, as previously discussed, in promoting optimal care.

Clear, Relevant, and Timely Communication Looking to the future of assisted living, many advocates stressed the importance of transparent information and disclosure to resident quality of life and care. They noted that incoming residents and their families often do not know what questions to ask about care, and that move in often occurs during an emotionally charged time; in consequence, they may sign contracts without understanding their full implications. Clear communication regarding service availability, costs, discharge policies, and other essential details can help consumers make well-informed decisions about their living arrangements, ensuring they understand their rights and options. Consumer advocates noted that this information must be communicated throughout the resident's stay, and that it must be explained in a way that is understandable to the resident and their support system:

> *"People need better information about what services are being provided, what's included in the base rate, what's a la carte, how much those costs are and who makes those determinations, what your rights are while you're there, what your rights are to stay, when can you be discharged, [whether there] are appeal rights … [we need] better communication throughout the process."*

The Provider Perspective

Upholding the Promise of Quality Providers acknowledged that even with the availability of thoughtfully developed tools and programs, not every assisted living community consistently delivers high-quality care. One provider recalled a personal experience with a family member who had Lewy body dementia:

> *"We [providers] all work really incredibly hard to create programs, trainings, supports, tools, so on and so forth, but I'll tell you in the real world where my brother-in law was a resident living with Lewy-body dementia in supposedly a really great memory care community, it was wildly disappointing. Even though they claim to do all those things, the real-world execution was so lacking, I was embarrassed on behalf of our industry to witness the really terrible care he received – and this is a place that promotes themselves as a great dementia provider."*

This experience underscored what many providers viewed as a promise that accompanies every resident's move in, saying *"I firmly believe we have a responsibility to deliver on that promise of really caring for them and supporting complex needs if that's what we said we're going to do."* To honor this commitment, providers stressed the importance of understanding the unique care environment of each community and achieving a strong person-environment fit. To the extent possible, doing so can be achieved by "staffing-up" to the care needs of residents, and recognizing when a community can no longer adequately support an individual's needs.

Third Parties and the Resident Experience Due to regulatory and community-based limitations on the type and extent of care available in assisted living, some residents and their support systems find it desirable to hire private duty caregivers. In discussing this phenomenon, providers remarked that while private duty caregivers can positively influence the resident experience, their qualifications vary widely, and can *"really create havoc in certain circumstances."* Providers noted that some communities have responded to this concern by hiring private duty "companions," individuals who are there for emotional support and may not perform personal care.

In addition to third-party caregivers, the relationship between providers, residents, and their families is fundamental to the overall care experience. Providers described navigating complex family dynamics, often fraught with emotion, and striving to provide support, education, and incorporate families into the resident's care. Said one provider, *"If we try to fragment what we do and focus solely on the resident, we're missing an opportunity. Families can be a real great partner with us but oftentimes they don't know what to expect or what we're able to do; we need to partner with them and educate them."*

Debating the Usefulness of the term "Quality of Life" When it comes to assessing care and resident experiences, many providers argued that the term "quality of life" is not appropriate for assisted living. One remarked, *"To me, "quality of life" is a SNF [skilled nursing facility] term; we shouldn't be using it in senior living."* Instead, providers proposed using "wellness" and "well-being" as the standard to measure resident outcomes, encouraging communities to recognize the interconnectedness of the varying types of social, supportive, and at times medical and mental health care provided by communities. Moreover, providers noted that the term "wellness," often defined as encompassing varying dimensions, better lends itself to practical applications than "quality of life." By defining wellness across specific dimensions, communities can design targeted programming; see Fig. 2 for specific examples provided by providers illustrating interventions related to four dimensions of wellness. As one provider noted, these simple yet effective programs

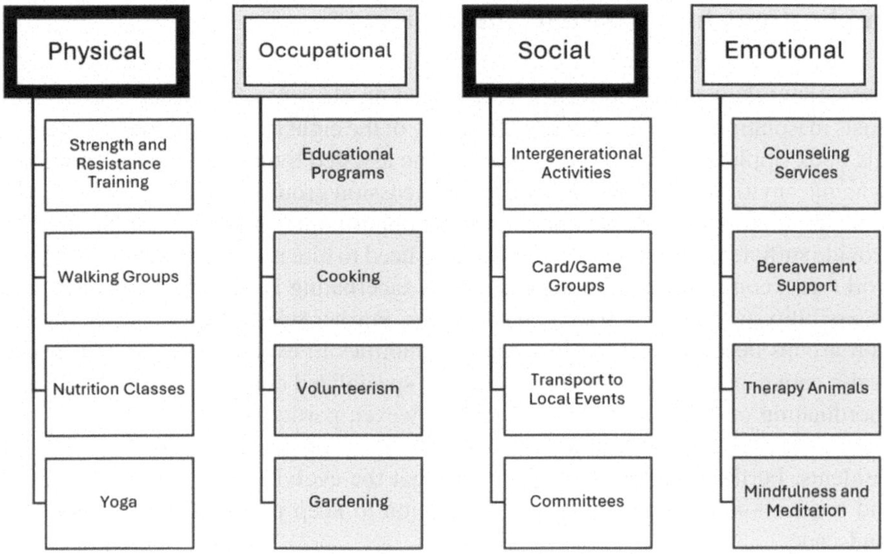

Fig. 2 Select interventions in assisted living based on dimensions of wellness

based on dimensions of wellness can potentially enhance residents' overall well-being. Additionally, targeted assessments of well-being can help residents articulate the support they need to live in accordance with what matters most to them.

Conclusion

Across provider and consumer advocate conversations, both groups shared many common perspectives on assisted living. Both reflected on the needs of individual residents in conjunction with staff capabilities and knowledge as defining the assisted living experience. Consumer advocates and providers discussed similarities and differences between assisted living communities and skilled nursing facilities and highlighted a shared recognition of the growing overlap between the services provided in assisted living and more traditional nursing home settings. While both groups acknowledged challenges—particularly surrounding affordability and the workforce—providers more frequently emphasized innovations and successes in providing person-centered assistance and care, while consumer advocates more often expressed concerns over gaps in clear communication and resident protections.

Implications for "Assisted" and "Living"

Throughout their discussions, it was clear that no element of "assisted" or "living" exists in isolation. Instead, changes across any of the eight topics explored throughout this book ripple across numerous facets of the assisted living experience, forming a dynamic environment. For example, both discussion groups noted that resident care needs have grown in complexity, presenting opportunities as well as challenges. To provide sufficient care, providers described a need to hire an increasingly specialized workforce, contributing to rising costs and exacerbating issues of affordability and accessibility, a concern shared by both groups. Further related to care needs, discussion groups described efforts in some communities to expand medical and mental health care capabilities, including providing specialized dementia care training and coordinating on-site end-of-life services; however, participants also acknowledged that care and the adequacy of training can fall short, compromising quality of life for residents. Furthermore, participants noted that the evolving needs of communities and residents necessitate changes in regulation to keep pace with an ever-shifting landscape.

The shared and occasionally divergent viewpoints of providers and consumer advocates illustrate a fundamental reality: among the tens of thousands of assisted living communities across the United States, some will succeed in delivering both "assistance" and "living," while others inevitably fall short. Some communities, guided by strong leadership and innovative strategies, successfully deliver high-quality care in a social environment responsive to residents' changing needs; others struggle with inconsistent regulatory enforcement, changing consumer expectations, and resource limitations, leading to service gaps that compromise both care quality and quality of life. Ultimately, the complexity of the challenges facing assisted living will require innovative and comprehensive solutions supported by rigorous research. Many such solutions, and related research, are detailed in previous chapters, while some are still waiting to be discovered.

Acknowledgments This chapter would not have been possible without the time and expertise of all discussion group participants: Rita Altman, Patrick Doyle, Gerald Hamilton, Bill Lamb, Sharon Roth Maguire, Kevin O'Neil, Doug Oliver, Kezia Scales, Lori Smetanka, Jennifer Svoboda, and Elizabeth H. Wheatley, whose insights and experiences are the foundation of its content. The authors additionally thank Kezia Scales for her thoughtful contributions to the framing of the chapter, and Esha Solanki for her assistance in strengthening its content and clarity.

Competing Interests The authors have no conflicts of interest to declare that are relevant to the content of this chapter.

References

1. Zimmerman S, Moczygemba W, Pace D, Laxton C, Schwartz L. Advancing excellence in assisted living: the evolution of CEAL@UNC. Caring Ages. 2025;26(2):17.
2. U.S. Department of Veterans Affairs. VA Aid and Attendance Benefits and Housebound Allowance [Internet]. 2024; cited 2025 Jul 25. https://www.va.gov/pension/aid-attendance-housebound/
3. Senior Lifestyle. How do Bridge Loans Work in Assisted Living Communities [Internet]. n.d.; cited 2025 Jul 25. https://www.seniorlifestyle.com/resources/blog/how-do-bridge-loans-work-in-assisted-living-communities/
4. Burns A, Wolk A, Watts MO, Mohamed M, Peña MTKFF. A look at waiting lists for Medicaid Home and Community-Based Services from 2016 to 2024. [Internet]. 2024; cited 2025 Oct 14. https://www.kff.org/medicaid/a-look-at-waiting-lists-for-medicaid-home-and-community-based-services-from-2016-to-2024/
5. CDC National Center for Health Statistics. Data from the National Post-acute and Long-term Care Study [Internet]. 2025; cited 2025 Jul 25. https://www.cdc.gov/nchs/npals/webtables/overview.htm
6. Centers for Medicare & Medicaid Services. Residents' Rights & Quality of Care [Internet]. 2025; Cited 2025 Jul 25. https://www.cms.gov/about-cms/what-we-do/nursing-homes/patients-caregivers/rights-quality-care
7. Centers for Medicare & Medicaid Services. Home & Community-Based Services 1915(c) [Internet]. 2025; Cited 2025 Jul 25. https://www.medicaid.gov/medicaid/home-community-based-services/home-community-based-services-authorities/home-community-based-services-1915c/index.html
8. Greene AM, Lepore M, Lux L, Porter K, Vreeland E. Understanding Unlicensed Care Homes: Final Report. 2015.; https://aspe.hhs.gov/reports/understanding-unlicensed-care-homes-final-report-0
9. National Center for Assisted Living. Assisted Living State Regulatory Review: 2023 Edition [Internet]. 2023; cited 2025 Oct 17. https://share.google/VKCxusZe47X90UIZH
10. Giardino AP, De Jesus O. Managed Care. [Updated 2022 Oct 24]. In: StatPearls [Internet]. Treasure Island (FL): StatPearls Publishing; 2025; cited 2025 Nov 16. https://www.ncbi.nlm.nih.gov/books/NBK564410/
11. Bridge Senior Living. Chamberlain University and Bridge Senior Living Launch Clinical Partnership to Introduce Nursing Students to Gerontology Field [Internet]. March 1, 2022 [cited 2025 Jul 25]. https://bridgeseniorliving.com/chamberlain-university-and-bridge-senior-living-launch-clinical-partnership-to-introduce-nursing-students-to-gerontology-field/
12. Zimmerman S. Balancing the equation: person-centered employment practices in assisted living. McKnight's Senior Living. 2024; https://www.mcknightsseniorliving.com/home/columns/guest-columns/balancing-the-equation-person-centered-employment-practices-in-assisted-living/
13. Pace D, Betts S, Reda L, Griff M, Stratton L, Shubeck E, Eichenberger L, Holles N, Holloway L, Little R, Maguire S, Mahoney J, Smith C, Fazio S. Empowering a person-centered long-term care workforce. Alzheimers Dement. 2024 Sep;20(9):6647–6653. doi:10.1002/alz.14111. Epub 2024 Jul 18. PMID: 39023198; PMCID: PMC11497762.
14. Bonvissuto K. Career ladders, lattices can provide opportunities, but there are issues: panel. McKnight's senior. Living. 2022; https://www.mcknightsseniorliving.com/news/career-ladders-lattice-can-provide-opportunities-but-there-are-issues-panel/
15. Zimmerman S, Sloane PD, Reed D. Dementia prevalence and care in assisted living. Health Aff (Millwood). 2014 Apr;33(4):658–66. https://doi.org/10.1377/hlthaff.2013.1255. PMID: 24711328
16. Zimmerman S, Williams CS, Reed PS, Boustani M, Preisser JS, Heck E, Sloane PD. Attitudes, stress, and satisfaction of staff who care for residents with dementia. Gerontologist. 2005 Oct;45 Spec No 1(1):96–105.

17. Hua CL, Cornell PY, Zimmerman S, Winfree J, Thomas KS. Trends in serious mental illness in US assisted living compared to nursing homes and the community: 2007-2017. Am J Geriatr Psychiatry. 2021 May;29(5):434–44. https://doi.org/10.1016/j.jagp.2020.09.011.
18. Provider Partners Health Plans. Institutional Equivalent Special Needs Plan (IE-SNP) [Internet]. n.d.; cited 2025 Nov 30. https://www.partnerwithpphp.com/ie-snp/
19. Centers for Medicare & Medicaid services. Guiding an Improved Dementia Experience (Guide) Model [Internet] 2025; cited 2025 Jul 25. https://www.cms.gov/priorities/innovation/innovation-models/guide

Index

H. Temkin-Greener and S. Zimmerman (eds.), *Assisted Living Through Research, Policy, and Practice*, https://doi.org/10.1007/978-3-032-32088-9

The manufacturer's authorised representative in the EU is Springer Nature Customer Service Centre GmbH, Europaplatz 3, 69115 Heidelberg, Germany. If you have any concerns regarding our products, please contact ProductSafety@springernature.com

Printed and bound by CPI Group (UK) Ltd, Croydon, CR0 4YY
21/09/2026
02220018-0006